15 LESSONS THAT CHANGED MY LIFE

Ashy Bines

15 LESSONS THAT CHANGED MY LIFE

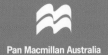

Pan Macmillan Australia

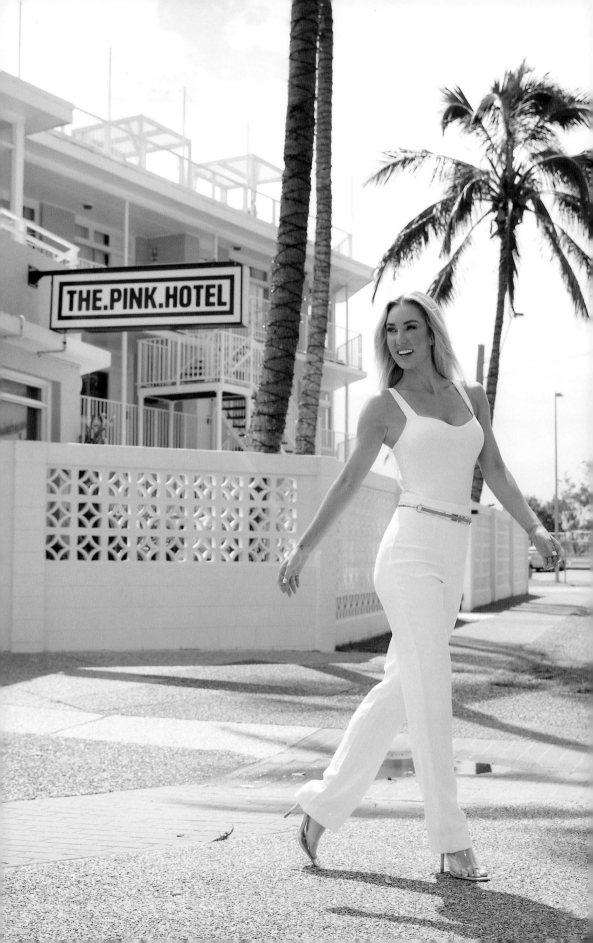

CONTENTS

Happiness

IS THE GOAL!

Wanting to make a difference to people's lives has been a constant for me for as long as I can remember. I never, ever want anyone feeling like they are alone, that no one cares, or for them to go through life just wishing it away.

All of us go through so many challenges and experiences in our lives that really can make or break us. We all also have a choice about what we do as a result of those experiences and challenges.

My mission is to help everyone, especially women, find happiness in their lives – and by that I don't mean through what someone's body looks like, but more importantly what's going on inside their minds. In no way does that mean I can give you the key to a perfect life, but I want us all to embrace and appreciate all the cards we get dealt in life, and find a way to use them to propel us forward in our lives.

The good moments should be celebrated and the harder times should be appreciated. Why, you ask? Because it's actually the most challenging times that offer us the opportunity to learn the most. Those moments force us to step up and grow. By growing we discover new ways to achieve, new ways to help others and ultimately it encourages us to set our own bar higher.

The good moments should be celebrated and the harder times should be appreciated.

When we can remember that life is happening FOR us, not TO us (thanks, Tony Robbins), we can navigate through life with way less pain and anxiety. It opens the door to bringing more excitement and joy into our day-to-day, no matter what kind of challenges we have to face.

Dissolving the fear and replacing it instead with real excitement for your day-to-day is what I am aiming to do. I truly believe the 15 life lessons in this book will help you so much across so many different areas of your life.

So, let's dive deep, let's open up, let's learn new ways of thinking and doing, so we can all feel more fulfilled, contribute to those around us and ultimately find more happiness.

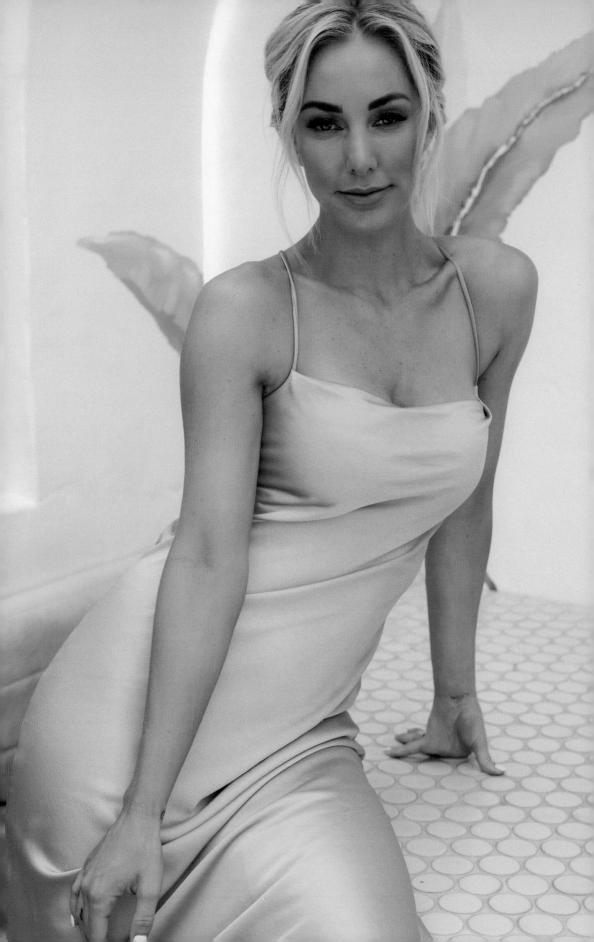

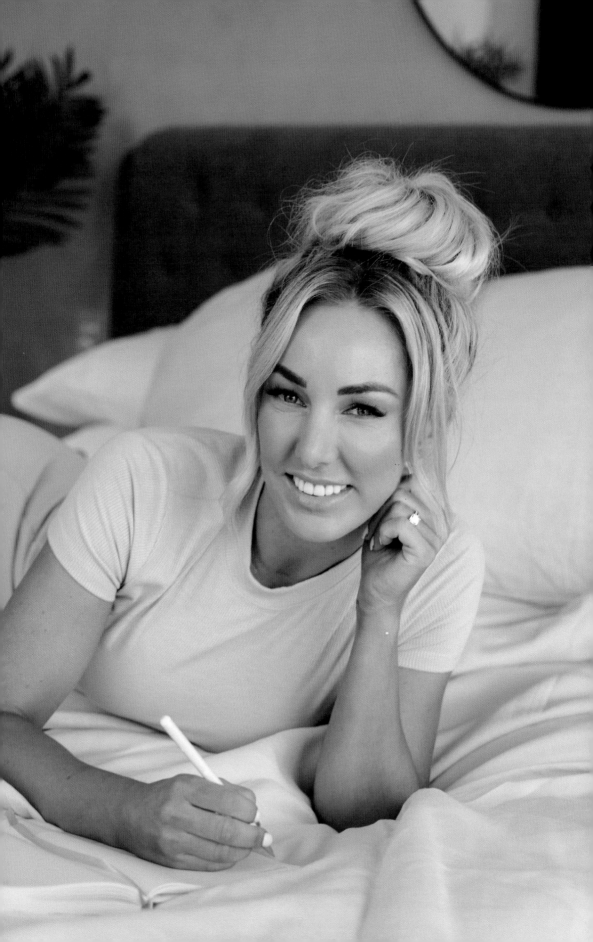

LESSON *One*

♥

Gratitude changes
everything

YOU CAN'T BE
ANGRY &

grateful

AT THE
SAME TIME

For years when I'd hear people say, 'Just be grateful', I would roll my eyes and think, 'Oh well, that's easy enough for YOU to say!' In hindsight, I now realise I didn't really understand the concept of gratitude well enough to live it, let alone practise it. I think you'd agree that gratitude is not something that comes naturally to many of us.

I hate to admit it, but I was always that Negative Nancy, constantly finding something to be angry about. I'm pretty sure some of you reading this are nodding your head and can totally relate. But let's face it – that kind of attitude doesn't make us feel happy, does it?

*So what if I told you that
our MINDSET can change
– but for that to happen,
WE need to change?*

If we are really serious about wanting anything to change in our lives, the only person who can create that change is US. Absolutely no one is going to do this for us. No one has a magic wand, and no one is going to come and save us. The reality is that WE need to start being our own hero.

Why does it often take something tragic, very challenging or sad to make us really feel grateful for the basic things in life? Have you ever lost something or someone and found that it really 'wakes you up' to the realisation that we just can't take things for granted?

I don't want dramatic events to shock me into feeling pure gratitude for everyone and everything. Ultimately, my goal is to always feel so very grateful.

From the age of 16, I was out of home and responsible for looking after myself. Managing basic things, like having enough money to put just enough fuel in my car to get me to and from work, was such a stress. Today, when I fill up at the petrol station, and I mean fully fill the tank – not just quarter- or half-fill it like I used to – I still remember when it wasn't this easy. I am proud of what I have achieved, because it means that I no longer have to stress about the basic things most of us take for granted.

> *I look back and am actually*
> *so grateful for those stressful times where*
> *I had to struggle because, hard as it was,*
> *it really did teach me gratitude. It also made*
> *me an extremely hard worker, so I also owe*
> *my work ethic to those lean times.*

Growing up, my biological father was not a part of my life, and I was always so jealous and almost bitter that my friends had such beautiful dads. Over time, I've flipped the resentment into gratitude that I have my mum, who I adore. Some people have zero family. Some never get to meet their biological mum or dad, and sadly some lose their parents to tragic accidents or illness. How lucky am I to still have my mum here. I am so very grateful for this and never, ever take it for granted.

Life really does teach us so much about being grateful. Before I became a mum, I didn't appreciate my body much at all. I was way more concerned about wanting it to look a certain way, rather than caring about what it was capable of doing – creating a human! Having to confront loss and illness in my close circle of friends and family also reinforced this new appreciation I had for my body. Losing my Pop to cancer and watching a good friend of a similar age to me battling cancer made me grateful for my health and for how well my body functions every single day.

Most of us really do just take for granted that we have two feet and a heartbeat. Think about it for a moment. Think about all the complex things all of our organs do, 24/7. Our heart beats 100,000 times a day – and we rarely even think about it. Our bodies are just incredible!

Increasingly, I am also so appreciative of my online audience who support me in all of my passions. Most of all, I'm so deeply grateful I have a voice that can help to inspire, motivate and create change. When I wrote this chapter, there were many bushfires burning across so much of Australia. I was overwhelmed with gratitude as I realised I could leverage my social media platforms to mobilise an online community and make a real difference to the people who have been impacted by the large-scale devastation of the fires. Together, we raised about $41,000 to help support those in need.

> *There is so much to be grateful for, everywhere*
> *we look – if we choose to open our eyes,*
> *minds and hearts.*

Stop for a moment, focus inwards and I know you'll agree. I want you to think about how most of us go about our day-to-day lives – getting out of our comfortable beds, scrolling through our social media, going to the gym or for a walk, kissing our loved ones good morning, deciding what to have for breakfast, hopping in our car or local transport, working at our jobs, catching up with friends, enjoying a hot bath and a nice dinner, watching some Netflix and maybe reading a page of this book. You're probably thinking, 'Yeah, sure, that's what I do most days – no big deal.' But, actually we need to just stop, take a breath and realise just how damn lucky we are to have all of this – ALL of it!

Gratitude

IS THE BEST
ATTITUDE

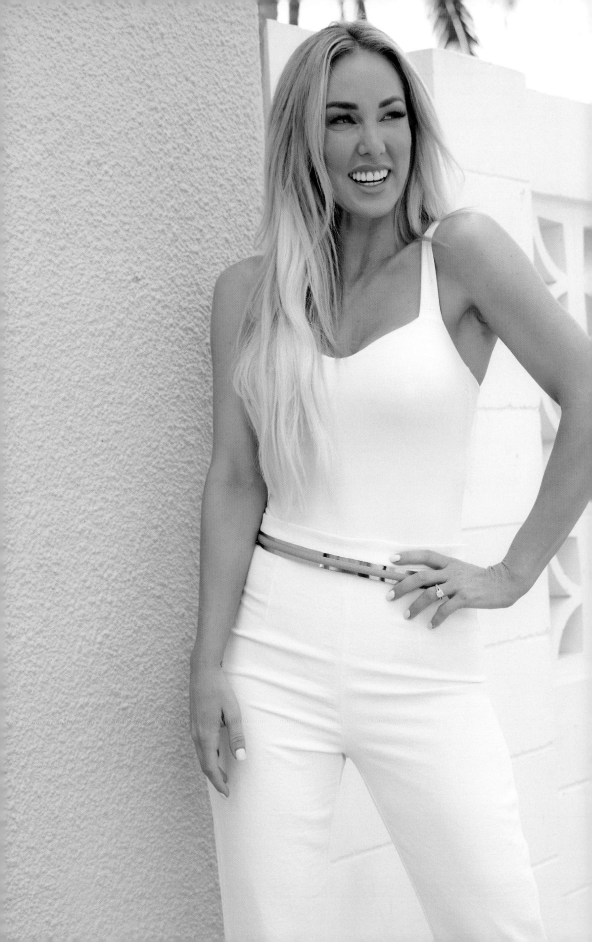

So many people around the world don't have clean water to drink or water to wash themselves or their clothes. They also don't know where their next meal is coming from or if and when they will see their loved ones again. They either don't have jobs or are forced to work in jobs they hate. They have no opportunity, no freedom and no choice. Yet we all get to complain about the weather, spilling our coffee or having to wait in line for a few more minutes than yesterday. Literally, First World Problems that don't deserve a mention.

It was important to me to start with this lesson as the first lesson in this book, as I cannot emphasise enough how really critical it is for us to not take anything, anyone or any single day for granted. None of us knows what tomorrow will bring, so let's try to embrace each and every day as if it were our last.

Even during the tough times, try hard to find appreciation and gratitude in the lessons these challenging moments are teaching us and the strength and growth they are giving us.

I know it can sometimes seem a little 'airy-fairy' or 'spiritual' – but honestly, this mindset of living in gratitude doesn't take much to learn and practise. Gratitude really is a key to building happiness.

HERE ARE MY TIPS TO GET YOU STARTED ON THE GRATITUDE JOURNEY

 When you wake up in the morning, please DON'T start your day scrolling your Instagram and comparing yourself to everyone's curated, 'picture-perfect' photos of their 'perfect' lives, relationships, jobs, bodies, etc.

 INSTEAD, sit up and take 10 deep breaths. Get yourself a gratitude journal or a notebook and jot down something – anything – that you are grateful for in your life.

 I aim to write three things each day, but sometimes it's just one and other days it's 10. But EVERY SINGLE DAY, there is something for us to be grateful for, and when we start our day grounded and grateful, it absolutely does set up the energy and vibe for the rest of our day.

 We can all agree that it's just way better to be around someone who is grateful, happy and light, rather than negative and complaining about everything. Who do you want to surround yourself with – and most importantly, who do YOU want to be?

THINGS TO

be grateful

FOR, RIGHT
NOW!

Don't forget to take 10 big breaths and REALLY focus
deeply about what you're grateful for in your life

1

2

3

4

5

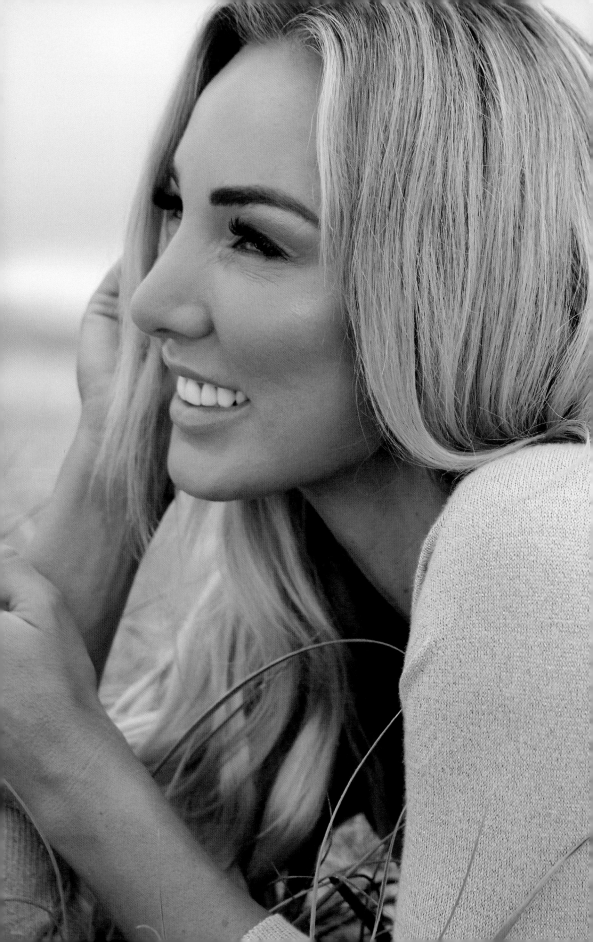

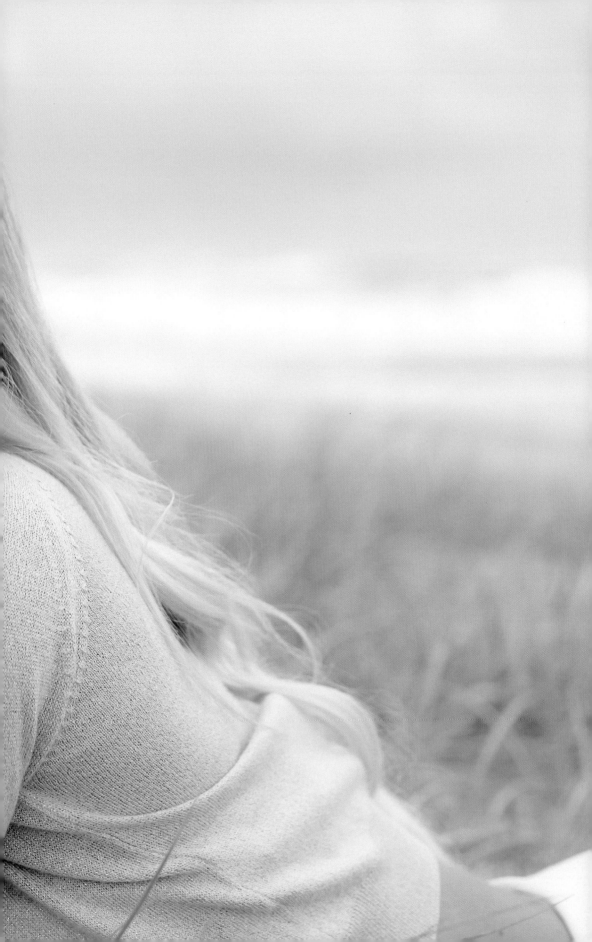

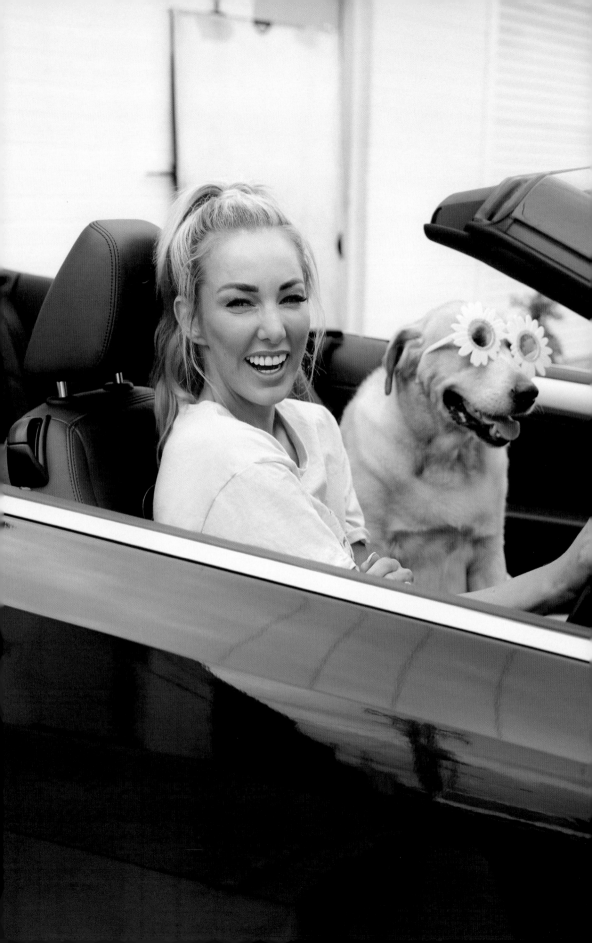

LESSON *two*

♥

You are not defined by your problems, you are defined by your response

YOUR STRUGGLES ARE
NOT WHO YOU ARE
BUT THEY CAN HELP
SHAPE WHO YOU
become

How do you view yourself and describe who you are? Has someone ever called you a name or suggested there is some-thing wrong with you? Has that negativity stuck with you, so you now see yourself in that way?

Do you find yourself constantly putting yourself down, calling yourself names or questioning if there's something wrong with you?

Pause for a moment and ask yourself if these thoughts are actually true. As in, are they *factually* correct? Or are you just twisting and bending the truth? Is this just a limiting belief and storyline that you are replaying on repeat in your own head?

We need to be super-vigilant and so aware of the stories we tell ourselves and the way we speak to ourselves, including the language we use. Because you better believe that everything our mind says, our body feels.

Having a flawed idea of who you are can cause a lot of anxiety, stress and unnecessary pain – and it can totally and absolutely hold you back in every part of your life.

I watched my mum and stepfather go through a divorce that emotionally really shook me up. I didn't have any idea how to cope or deal with it all. I just wanted to be strong for my mum, and for a long time I tried doing exactly that – but, internally, I wasn't dealing with my own emotions. I felt paralysed in a state of hopelessness and wasn't able to move through what had happened. In the end, I just couldn't wrap my head around how much it was hurting my mum – and I took all of that on myself.

It wasn't just how I was feeling on the inside. I would be shaking constantly, having panic attacks, crying every day, ripping my hair out and not sleeping, and I would go days without eating. It was relentless. I was in a constant 24/7 state of anxiety.

Friends who could see what I was going through and the damage it was causing told me I needed help and urged me to see a doctor. Eventually, I took their advice.

The consultation with the doctor was a very brief 15 minutes. He told me I was depressed and diagnosed me with anxiety. He wrote a prescription for some medication and sent me home. That was it – nothing more.

At no point did he want to know if I was okay or what was causing me to feel anxious or depressed. He also didn't offer any kind of solution except the medication. Looking back, I wish he had said something, anything, constructive or helpful – even if he had just reminded me to breathe. But I got nothing. I was sent away with no guidance, no support and feeling as helpless and distressed as when I'd arrived.

From that moment, if anyone had asked me to describe who 'Ashy Bines' was, I would have replied, 'She's anxious and depressed.' I had allowed the doctor's words during that very rushed assessment to completely and utterly define me – but it wasn't who I was at my core.

If you are reading this and are feeling the same or if you have let someone else's words define you, then I'm here to tell you – no, that is NOT who you are!

I took the doctor's advice and took medication for my depression and anxiety for almost a year. It was only after going to my first Tony Robbins course that I decided it was time to come off the medication and face whatever was going to come up, lean into the old wounds and unpack the old stories. It is important to talk to your doctor before coming off medication.

Every single day I feel excited and passionate about the projects, concepts and ideas I'm working on. But it wasn't always like that.

It was time to stop playing the victim and instead try to find a new and more empowering meaning to what had happened in my past.

Now, I'd be lying if I told you that I no longer experience any anxiety. Yes, I still do. However, today I have so many more tools and so much more support around me, so that when these feelings emerge, I am in a much better position to manage them. I'm really not sure if I'll ever truly be able to say that I no longer get anxious – but I'm continually learning new ways to deal with it. Today, I'm also far kinder to myself and no longer try to bury my true feelings. This is also the reason why self-care is such a crucially important part of my life.

So, I want you to make a list of all the AMAZING qualities YOU have as a person.

Of course it's okay if right now you are feeling anxious, sad, angry or are going through a hard time, but let's focus on the beautiful qualities that you have and that are a part of who you really are. Be proud of all the amazing things you are – so let's push those qualities to front of mind!

It's time to start labelling yourself with the positive stuff, not the things that don't feel good in your heart, in your head or in your body.

Every single one of us – whether we are parents, sisters, aunts or friends – has to remember that the more work we do on ourselves and our old wounds from past experiences helps us to grow and develop in a positive way. Remember, too, that our own personal growth is not limited to ourselves, but has a strong ripple effect on our kids, our families, our friends and pretty much everyone we come into contact with in our lives.

WHAT QUALITIES DO YOU LOVE IN YOURSELF?

These examples are the qualities I love in myself and also the ones I want to get better at being. Fill in the rest of the spaces with qualities that are important to you.

♥ | Playful

♥ | A good listener

♥ | Funny

♥ | Selfless

♥ | Sensual

♥ | Bubbly

♥ | Generous

♥ | Cuddly

♥ | Hard-working

♥ |

♥ |

♥ |

♥ |

♥ |

This realisation was really brought home to me after becoming a mum. Having a family has been a real motivator for me to continue working on myself. My hope is for my children to grow up being proud of who they are and to have the confidence to work through whatever challenges and issues they may face in life. I never want them to be defined by anyone else's view of them. I want my children to be comfortable being true to themselves.

Your struggles are NOT who you are –
but they can help shape who you become.
Remember, you get to choose.

Being true to yourself is everything. It took me a long time to get to that point and that's why I'm sharing my experiences – in the hope that it might help make the journey easier for you.

We just can't live our lives pleasing others at the cost of our own happiness and energy.

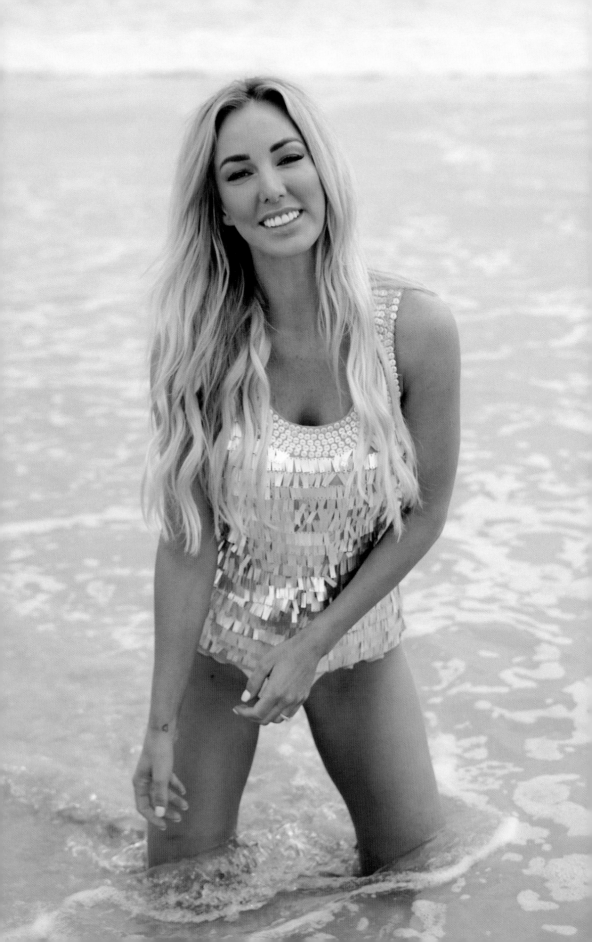

TOO MANY
OF US ARE NOT
LIVING OUR
dreams
BECAUSE WE
ARE LIVING
OUR FEARS

Ask your three closest friends to write in here and _describe you_, you might be very surprised!

_____

_____

_____

_____

_____

Ask your friends to also make a list of _what they love about themselves_. And you, too, can add _what you love about them._

_____

_____

_____

_____

_____

This should give each of you all of the feels!

Commit to doing this more often in your life. Highlighting those things to someone else might just help them see themselves in a more positive way.

AT THE VERY LEAST,
YOU'LL MAKE THEIR DAY!

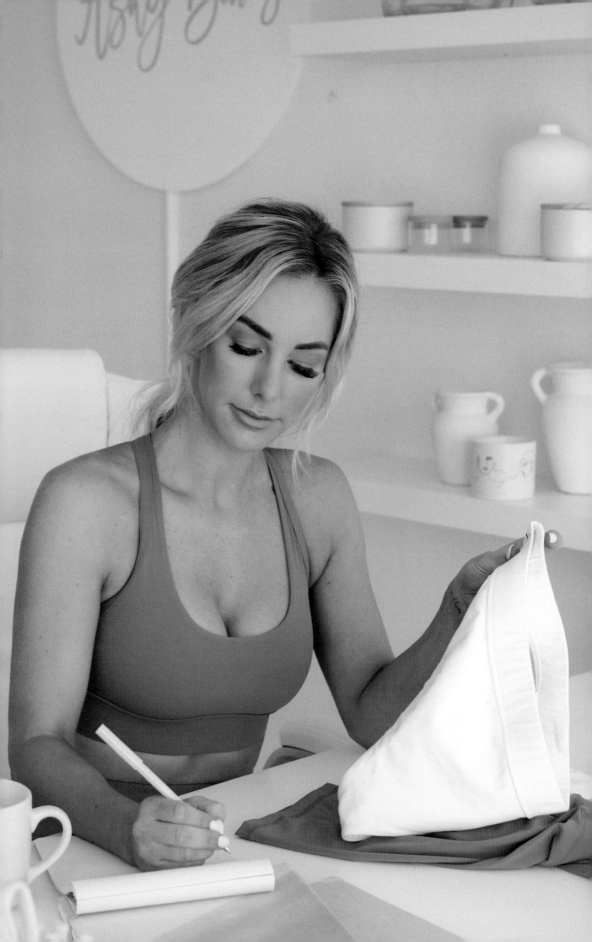

LESSON *Three*

♥

Find passion in relationships, work and life

FOLLOW YOUR
PASSION. IT WILL
LEAD YOU TO YOUR

purpose

Oprah Winfrey

Did you wake up this morning excited about your day or the person you're lying next to or knowing you'll be seeing someone you think is amazing or just feeling happy about the day you've planned?

Or, are you reading this thinking 'Hell no. That's definitely not how I'm feeling – at all'?

Don't panic! Just remember, things can change, if we decide to make the change.

It's so, so easy to get stuck in a routine and just go about our daily lives in autopilot, without giving it much thought. Very soon, that becomes our normal and in our minds we feel trapped by the routine, believing we don't have any choice and it's just something 'we have to do'. Right?

Well, I absolutely 100 per cent disagree!

WE ALL HAVE CHOICES:

WHAT we do

WHO we do it with

HOW often we do things

WHEN we do them

WHERE they happen

What I am definitely not saying is if you're unhappy, just go quit your job today. We all have responsibilities and bills to pay. Yes, I totally get that some of you may not be enjoying what you're doing right now or that you see it as a stepping stone to get to where you eventually want to be… but this chapter is a reminder for you to check in with yourself to see how happy you really feel. It's also an opportunity to reconnect with that word: 'PASSION'.

Our aim is to find passion in everything we do!

Many years ago, I actually believed 'passion' was something only the 'lucky people' got to experience in their work, their relationships and in their lives. I truly thought 'passion' bypassed everyday regular people like me. Oh hello, 'victim mentality', we meet again! Excuse me for that lapse… Growing up, I was a massive victim – but that's another entire chapter in itself. ;-)

Passion is absolutely something that everyone deserves, and you can build it into your life! Now, I'm not talking about some fleeting, temporary moment of passion – I mean something you can create and grow across all parts of your life. I want you to live your passions.

LET'S START WITH RELATIONSHIPS

I'd say most people would agree that it's so very easy to get lazy and comfortable in a marriage or partnership. My beautiful husband, Steve, and I have been together for just over 10 years and I'm not afraid to admit that there have been times when we have lost our passion for each other. Let me also be the first to tell you that, boy, that situation does not feel nice!

Our relationship moved pretty fast and we had some really tough life challenges thrown our way quite early on, so we didn't get much of a honeymoon stage. More recently, we've become more awake, conscious and aware about our relationship and can recognise when we get lazy or don't put each other's needs first. When we don't stay connected, we can feel that distant energy and it's not a place we want to stay in for long.

Relationships take a lot of work, commitment, love and understanding – and I truly believe that if both people are on a growth journey, together you can push through anything.

I don't live in some fairytale believing that nothing could ever, ever break us. Let's be real, we never know what the future holds – but what I do know is when there is love, understanding, compassion and really clear, great communication, it's a beautiful partnership and such a fun journey. Now that's relationship goals! We're so grateful for our partnership, which is so much more than just a cute smoochy photo on the internet. The thing we both love in each other is the commitment we each invest in working together on whatever life throws at us.

Sure, we've had confronting moments in our marriage where we've scrambled to find answers – asking ourselves, is there something wrong with us? Were we even meant to be together? It took time and work to figure out that it was none of the above. Eventually, we came to the realisation that maintaining the passion in our lives was like anything in life: if you want to feel and live a passionate life, only you can make it happen!

There is no secret to share or magic pill you can take. It's all about getting to know what lights us up on the inside. What makes us feel excited and joyful when we do certain activities or are around certain people. It's about the energy we bring into our relationships or lives every single day.

*If you want to feel and live a passionate life,
only YOU can make it happen!*

Steve and I prioritise working on our relationship so that we keep that passion alive. We believe in date nights and think they should be a forever thing! The longer you're together as a couple, the more important it is to have date nights, so that you can focus on each other and your feelings rather than the usual day-to-day stuff. Becoming parents has made it even more important to schedule in our date nights where we can connect with each other again, one on one.

Understanding and always being aware and conscious of each other's love languages and human needs is important for our relationship.

THE FIVE LOVE LANGUAGES

Words of affirmation

Acts of service

Quality time

Receiving gifts

Physical touch

Every single one of us has a way we express love and affection, and a way we like to receive love and affection. Not recognising these can have real impacts on our relationships and things can break down. It can mean that you or your partner may not be feeling loved despite your best efforts, purely because the way you're giving love is not how they feel it.

To help you understand and relate, let's look at Steve and me as an example. Steve's main love language is physical touch. He loves intimacy, holding hands, cuddling 24/7, hands resting on legs at tables, kissing – basically anything where I'm physically touching him. For me, physical touch is maybe third on my list. The main way I feel love is acts of service. So, when Steve does something for me, I get that feeling of 'Awwww wow, that's so nice and I feel all filled up inside!' But it can be challenging for both of us – because acts of service don't come naturally to him and I'm not naturally a super-touchy person. So, ensuring we both feel loved really does mean us being very aware, awake and conscious to the other person's love language, otherwise they are going to feel very unloved. There is an entire book about this by Gary Chapman, called *The Five Love Languages*, and I highly recommend it!

Surprising each other often is something we still ensure we do. Variety and spicing up life is so important. Go ahead and be playful and don't forget about the things you used to do when you first became a couple. Steve and I try so hard to not just get caught up in the 24/7 routine of day-to-day work, stress and parenting. It's too easy to let yourself slip into a rut, and then life can become mundane and maybe even boring. Personally, that's not what I aspire to – I always want to push myself to feel and live passionately, because passion is frigging AMAZING.

Little gestures count, like holding hands in the car, sending a flirty text, leaving little love notes around, a random act of kindness or just letting your loved one know what you appreciate about them, often.

How much do you love it when your partner does these nice cute things? How much does it light you up and spark that passion again? Well … GET ON IT, GIRL!

Life coach and motivational speaker Tony Robbins has always been one of the biggest inspirations in my life. He encourages us to live life to the fullest, to work through our challenges and to own them and take responsibility for them. During one of his seminars I attended, he shared some solid advice on relationships that really resonated with me. He said, 'Do what you did at the start of your relationship at the end – and there won't ever be an end.'

And that is truth!

Now, before anyone twists my words, of course I understand that sometimes relationships don't work. And that's okay, because let's face it, everyone's situations are very different and things do happen. Sometimes we grow apart from our partners, fall out of love or just want different things. However, so many relationships break down from lack of understanding, lack of growth or connection or not being supportive enough of each other's triggers and traumas – and sometimes simply because of the lack of variety or passion.

Remember the start of your relationship, when it was always really fun, open, when there was loads of variety and adventure, great communication and passion? It made you feel alive, right? Those butterflies in your tummy and wanting to spend every single moment with that person… and nothing else even enters your mind because you're so in 'lust'? So at what point did that all evaporate, and when did it become okay to be just mediocre? Why can't we live passionately forever? Why can't we have those feelings always? Since when did it become cool to just settle? No thanks!

I'll say it again: just remember things can change, if we decide to make the change.

WHAT ABOUT PASSION IN OUR WORK LIVES?

Some of us find it easy to figure out what kind of work lights us up, but for others – like me, for example – it can take a little time and experimentation to find the work we love!

Have you ever added up how many hours you spend at work? If you have a regular nine-to-five, Monday-to-Friday job, that's about 40-plus hours a week. For many of us, it would actually be a lot more; for me, it's up to 60 hours a week. But in any given week I probably wouldn't be able to tell you how many hours I've worked that week, because most of the time it doesn't feel like work!

Every single day I feel excited and passionate about the projects, concepts and ideas I'm working on. But it wasn't always like that.

Back in the day, I worked in jobs I hated. And I mean hated from the moment I woke up with that feeling of dread or actual anxiety that I had to get up and go to work. Once at work, I would literally count down the hours to my lunch break, and then after lunch I'd be counting down the hours until I could finally run out the door. I would race back home to binge-watch TV, because all I wanted to do was escape my reality. What a way to live, right? That was not living – it was surviving.

It impacted every part of my life. My mental state, my moods and even what I ate. Feeling so desperately unhappy and unfulfilled meant I stopped caring about my health and my body. Suppressing and numbing my feelings with distractions like TV and unhealthy food was my way of coping.

I had no direction, no passion. In fact, I just felt dead inside.

In those times, we absolutely have to ask ourselves: are we thriving or just surviving?

Life is way too short and I don't want to merely survive each day.

We often forget how insanely lucky we are to be here and the amazing freedom of choice we have available to us.

There are many people in other countries and cultures that have zero choice and would be grateful to be in our position. So why are we settling? You want more? Great! Guess what? You can have more!

I know, I know, people say, 'Just follow your passion'. I know this word can be overused and you can get sick of hearing it from everyone you follow on social media.

So you may be reading this feeling pretty down, not feeling that you are at a point in your life where you are living your life passionately. Or you may not even know what your passion is yet. That is totally okay! Sometimes it can take a little time and more self-discovery, and our passions can also change and evolve as we grow or go through life. That's all a part of the journey, too.

Look at my mum's experience. She started off as a dairy farmer, then became a school teacher and finally landed in finance because Mum is really smart and really good with numbers. She stayed in that finance job until she was 52 years old because numbers were her strength and she needed to pay the bills and feed her family. Fair enough, right?

No– wrong.

Well, yes, she did have us kids to feed and bills to pay, but it was her choice to stay there for so long.

Then one day, in a random moment, she tried making soap at home and BOOM! Not only did she realise she was super creative and talented when it comes to making soap, but wow, she was really passionate about soap!

She began making soap in her kitchen and selling a few online – and BOOM five years later it's turned into a huge company. In fact, it grew into such a big operation that she needed to focus more of her time on running the business side of things, rather than doing the creative – which is what she was passionate about in the first place! So Mum decided to sell the business to me and Steve because we are passionate about running businesses and wanted to continue the legacy she had created.

The greatest thing Mum learned was that despite being great with numbers, that side of business just makes her feel dead inside. She refused to do a job she didn't feel passionate about. I love that my mum found a way to have the freedom and space to focus on her creative side and immerse herself in projects that make her feel alive! Her story is abso-lute proof that passion can create magic!

There is ALWAYS a solution –
it's just finding the right path.

Once you've found the thing that lights you up, you just need to start figuring out how you can make it part of your life. Please don't try to do everything at once and make it too overwhelming.

Just start with one thing at a time, and try to find some space in your life over the next few weeks to include them. Once you've done that, it's time to explore ways that you can turn what you're passionate about into a real career.

If you're feeling stuck and unsure what you're passionate about, I encourage you to take a moment to make a list of the things you enjoy.

For me, health and fitness were things I truly loved, but I was also always so deeply passionate about wanting to help people to not feel alone. Being a supportive person, a good listener and always being there to help others was something that really resonated with me and reflected who I was on a deep level. Becoming a personal fitness trainer was that incredible moment in my life when I realised that I could combine my two passions in life and make a real impact. It has turned into something way bigger than I'd ever dreamed.

This new life allowed me so many things that I had been craving: flexibility, working for myself and the chance to train outdoors in the fresh air and by the ocean, which I adore. It gave me access to financial opportunities, a variety of clients with different goals and unique personalities, a schedule that I could control, time for my friends and family and time to develop exciting projects within my business. It was both exciting and challenging and I was never bored! Importantly, I was doing exactly what I loved doing and being true to who I was while making a real difference and positive changes to people's lives, not just physically, but also mentally and emotionally. I was living my passion and my purpose – and I still do! When you love what you do, it never gets tired. I want each of you to experience that, too!

Remember, even if you can't make a career based on your passion, I want you to think about how you can still embrace it. How often can you engage with that passion? Work on that passion? Share that passion? Make passion a true focus and priority in your life.

Make it your mission in life not merely to
SURVIVE but to THRIVE.

REMEMBER THE
FOUR 'P' WORDS

Finding **Passion**
and living **Passionately**

Having a strong **Purpose** and
sense of why in your life

Believing in your own **Power** to
create the life you truly want

Finding the **Positives** and gifts
in all situations

Passion, Purpose, Power, Positivity

Make a list of what you LOVE doing

_____

_____

_____

_____

Make a list of what you HATE doing

_____

_____

_____

_____

Ask yourself, which job would you do for a year and
not even worry about getting paid? Or, if money wasn't
an issue, what job would you love to do?

_____

_____

_____

_____

Now ask your three closest friends the same questions.

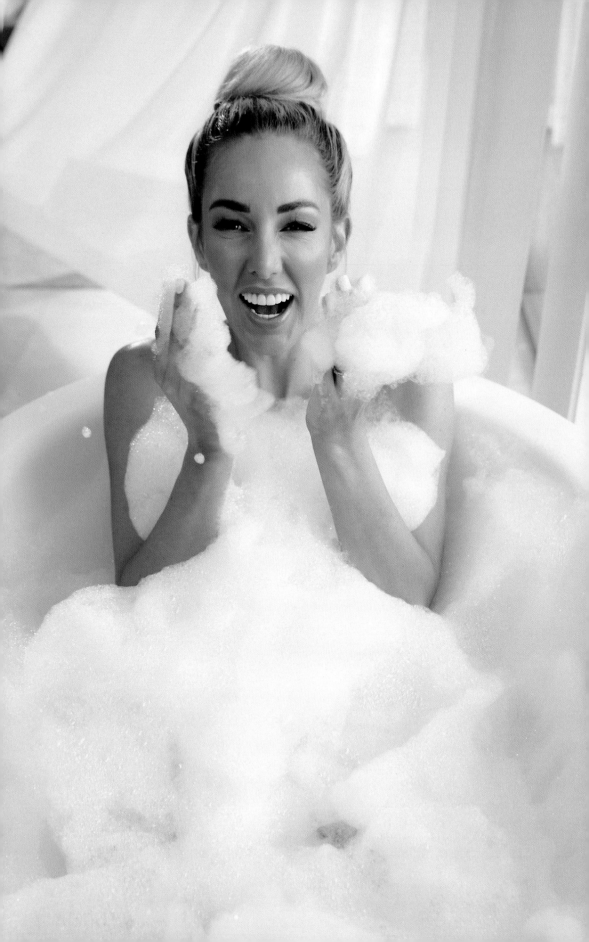

LESSON *Four*

♥

Don't be a people pleaser

DON'T BE AFRAID
TO LOSE PEOPLE
BE AFRAID OF
LOSING

yourself

BY TRYING TO
PLEASE EVERYONE
AROUND YOU

Do you never say what you want? Offer to do things you don't want to do? Always fit in with everyone else's schedule's? Never put up your hand to ask for help? Do you have a real hunger for approval and just want to avoid conflict at all costs?

If you answered YES to most or all of the questions above, then there's a pretty good chance you're a People Pleaser.

Now, I am certainly not judging. I was – and sometimes still am – a People Pleaser, too!

Yes, it's human for us to want to be liked and accepted – but is that okay if it means not being true to ourselves and having to sacrifice our identity along the way?

Being so eager to please people can be due to many different reasons, but for me – and, I believe, so many others – it can come from how I view myself and, more specifically, my issues about my own self-worth.

This is something in my life that I am still working on all the time. But I'm increasingly very aware of lapsing into People Pleaser mode and now catch myself way more often. I've also learned that there are times when I am definitely more vulnerable to falling back into the people-pleasing habit. When I'm feeling drained or exhausted, I know that I have to mentally check in with myself and review the things I may have agreed to take on, that in reality I really didn't want to do – or couldn't really fit into my schedule or life.

I've come to understand that I'm the type of person who wants to help, but at the same time also very much wants to be liked. I now recognise that this comes from a deeper sense of insecurity about not feeling that I am 'enough'.

Growing up, I never really felt like I was enough for anyone. I never felt good enough, smart enough or funny enough. To compensate for everything I thought I was lacking, I would automatically say 'yes' to everything, just to please people. In my mind, I thought agreeing to help with everything would make everyone love me more, and I would feel more loved.

But is that what we really want?

The thing I believe we really want, crave, and totally deserve is for people to appreciate and love who we are as a person! Let's never forget that each one of us is an amazing and unique individual. Those who truly do love us will not only love us for being brave enough and strong enough to stand in our power and with kindness say 'no' – but they will also respect us for it!

I know some of you are reading this, still thinking how stressful it is to say 'no' and that's why you don't do it – and can't even imagine doing it! You're thinking, 'I don't even know how to say NO!'

> *Do we want to be loved just because we*
> *are someone who says YES to everything,*
> *and does things for everyone?*

Communication, language and tone are critical when it comes to saying 'no'. Many of us struggle to say 'no', fearful someone won't like us or will be angry or get upset. It's all in the way we respond.

Ditch your fear and instead channel your kindness, is my advice.

If any of my friends were to say something like that to me, my response would probably be to go home and make them chicken soup and some 'clean treats'. Their honesty about how they are feeling actually makes me want to help them. I would never want them to feel bad for saying 'no' and choosing to look after themselves.

If the people around you are not being understanding of your own energy and needs, then maybe it's time for you to re-evaluate who you are surrounding yourself with and ask yourself if they deserve your time and energy.

Understanding and compassion are key foundations to maintaining healthy relationships with each other. Being comfortable saying 'no' – and also providing a safe space for people to be able to say 'no' to us – is going to build a much stronger connection between us all.

Haven't we all experienced times in our lives where we are no good to anyone, but we ignore this and still say 'yes' to everything, even when it doesn't feel right? Don't forget that the people around us are not mind-readers, and don't know how we are feeling unless we communicate it to them. We all need to recognise that it's really important to have boundaries, particularly when it comes to our energy and time. Let's face it, we can only really blame ourselves if we are feeling drained, used, exhausted and empty.

Yes, it can be a little scary to set those boundaries, and, yes, it takes guts – but once you do, then everything just has to fit around those boundaries. You are in charge of saying 'no'. We need to make the effort to learn how to self-soothe, to reserve energy and to include self-care in our lives. We also need to accept that this is a priority. Filling our own cup up is critical for our mental health and wellbeing.

HERE'S A WAY TO SAY NO THAT DOESN'T HURT YOU – OR THEM:

'Oh, I'd love to help you do that today, but if I'm being honest, I just feel so mentally, emotionally and physically exhausted. I really need to rest and organise my own chores, so I'm so sorry I'll have to say no today. Next time, when I'm feeling better, I can help you for sure.'

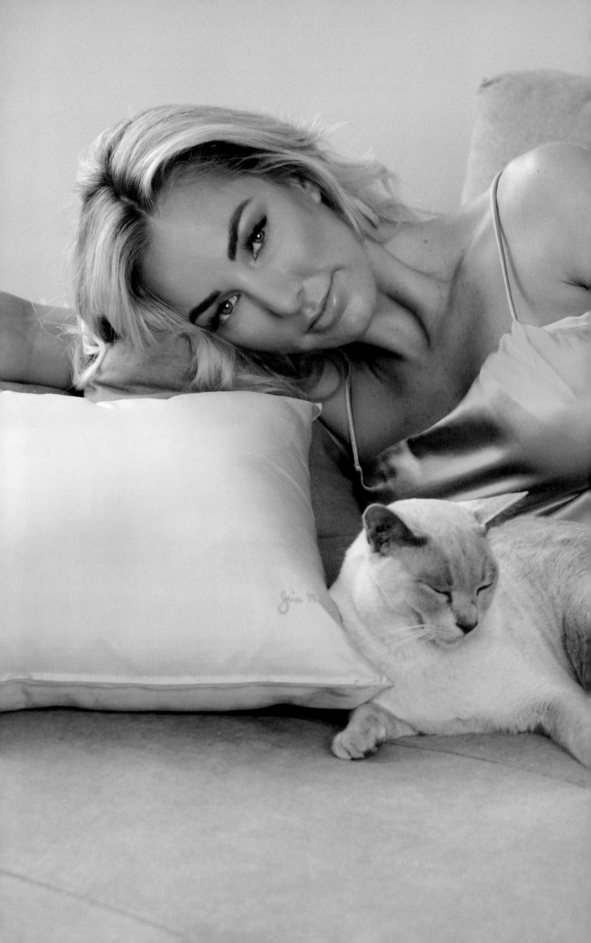

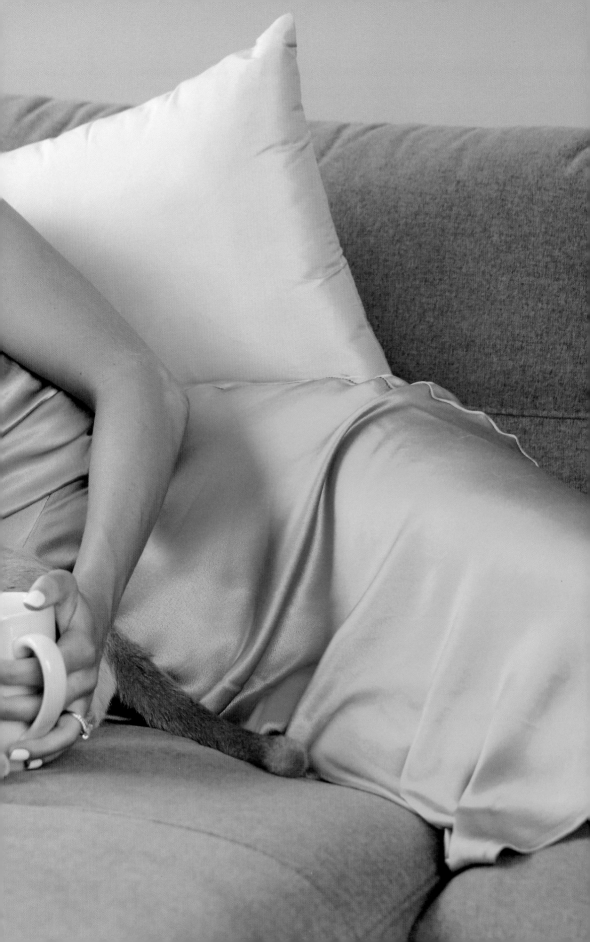

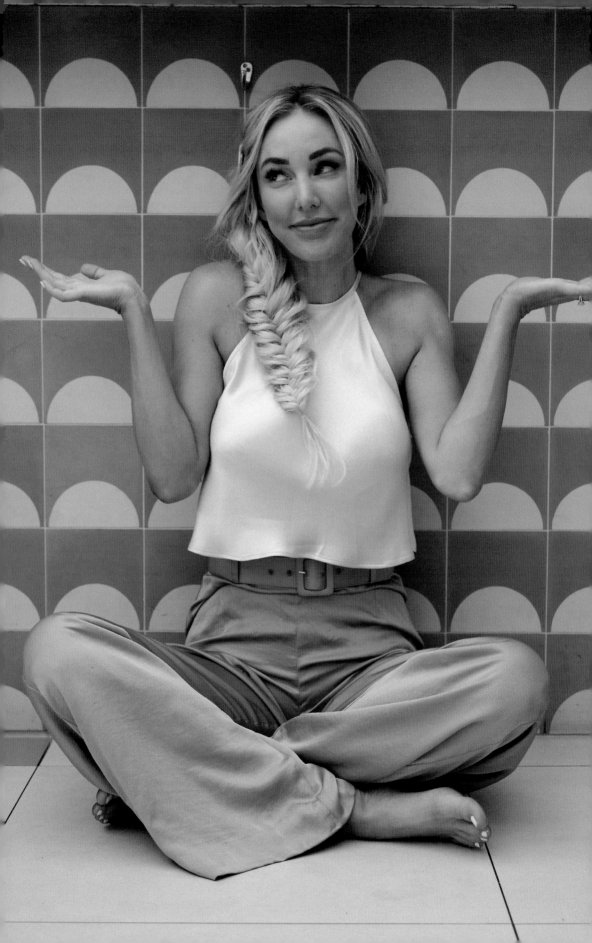

LESSON *Five*

♥

Don't blame. Take
responsibility for yourself
and your life

LIFE DOESN'T
HAPPEN TO YOU
IT HAPPENS

for you

This has got to be one of the hardest, and yet most rewarding, lessons I've learned in my life so far. And it's a lesson I still haven't quite nailed.

Yes, guilty!

I absolutely admit that I do sometimes have to catch myself and stop blaming someone else instead of owning it.

Why? Well, as we all know, it's way easier to blame – But do you realise that this is going to impact you emotionally in the long term? Pushing blame onto others places us in the position of … victim!

Taking on the role of victim can be the easy way out in the short term, but longer term it will be the very thing that holds us back from growth. Also, the victim mentality brings with it an energy that is really not that enjoyable to be around or attractive to other people.

It changes me. It makes me grumpy and sad, overly sensitive and irritable, and downright negative. This is absolutely the opposite of the positive, happy, inspiring energy that I want!

At one point when I was growing up, I had someone in my life who never missed an opportunity on the daily to tell me just how worthless and dumb I was, while also making sure to point out to me that I was a complete waste of space and not worthy of love. This person was 100 per cent certain I would never make anything of myself – and, eventually, I would 100 per cent believe every negative thing they said about me. Although I always had my mum's unwavering support, their words became my truth.

When I'm in a victim 'state of mind', I know for certain that I'm not allowing myself to be the best version of myself.

By my late teens, I was feeling very unloved and very unworthy. At a point in my life when I was looking to the future and starting to make decisions about my career path, all I felt was scared, confused and pretty much paralysed with self-doubt. I truly believed that I was too stupid and too dumb to have any kind of career in anything!

And I blamed this person for all of it!

It was all their fault that I felt sad and pathetic. It was all their fault, because of the way they treated me. It was all their fault that I was doing nothing with my life. It was all their fault that I was broke and depressed. It was all their fault that I was having constant panic attacks. Who I had become was all their fault. How I felt every day was all their fault.

It was all their fault – everything! No one else's fault, just theirs.

Were those stories TRUE? **NO**

Was it TRUE I was too dumb? **NO**

Was it TRUE I'd never be loved? **NO**

Things can and will happen to us throughout our lives. But we get to choose how it impacts us and changes us, for better or for worse.

How we view each experience and situation is in our hands. We get to choose if we become a victim or whether we use the hard times as opportunities to grow. Only we can decide to view them as gifts given to us in the form of a life lesson that will help us become wiser, emotionally stronger and mentally more resilient.

Navigating through challenging times and putting a positive meaning onto them helps us grow and learn. The benefits to our mental health, our lives and our emotional growth are undeniable. And how freaking inspiring do we also become to others? We now have better tools and more experience and compassion to help others around us to not feel alone when they, too, go through something difficult.

I'm not at all saying it's okay for people to mistreat us, because that's totally not okay in any situation. The way this person treated me was never okay, but I can't change the past. What I can do is find the gift, find the lessons and ultimately find gratitude in how it has shaped me to become so strong and resilient, and given me a strong fire in my belly to serve others and help them get through their own tough times.

THREE THINGS YOU NEED TO QUIT DOING NOW

1. Let's stop hating on
ourselves

2. Let's not blame others for
our problems

3. Let's start being grateful

*Remember – you can't be grateful
and angry at the same time*

TURNING A NEGATIVE INTO A POSITIVE

♥ | I really want you to take a moment to think about a situation that's happened in your life, where someone 'did' something that affected you in a really negative way.

♥ | Now, when you think back to this situation, take 10 massive breaths.

♥ | As hard as it is, ask yourself: how could you have done better? How could you have helped the situation?

♥ | Or, if there was truly nothing you could have done, instead of continuing to hate and blame the other person or situation, ask yourself: how did it CHANGE you? How much stronger has it made you?

♥ | Did it put you on a path that led you to meet new, amazing people?

♥ | Has it made you more compassionate? Has it made you more resilient?

♥ | Do you think the way you were treated showed you how NOT to treat people – and that's why you now treat others with kindness?

♥ | Did it make you a good listener? Did it make you more generous with your love and your time?

♥ | Although I don't know what you've experienced and been through, I do know that when we stop blaming and take responsibility instead, everything can CHANGE! If we dig really deep to find the lessons and growth in these situations, then we can find gratitude in almost everything.

♥ | Where do you want to live, emotionally?

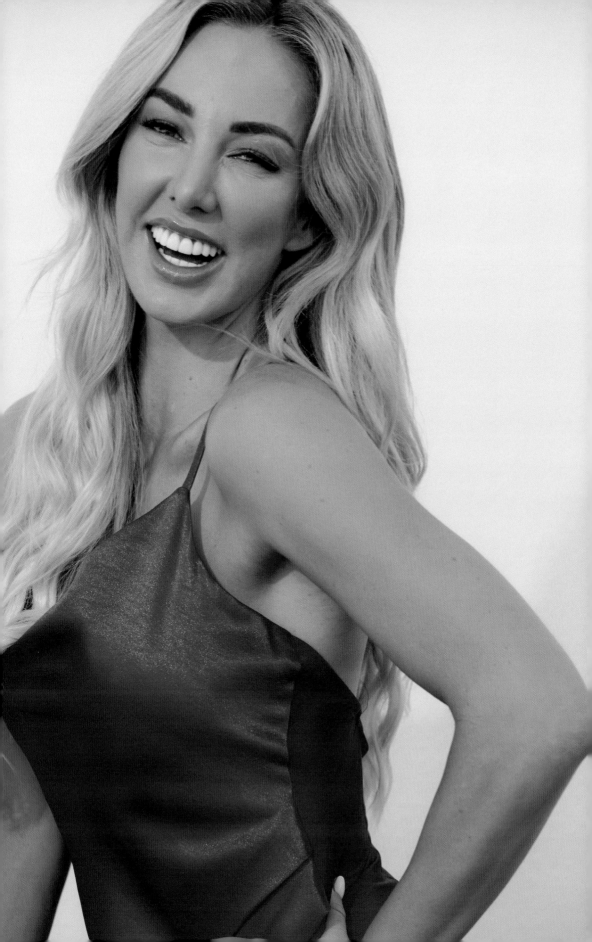

LESSON *Six*

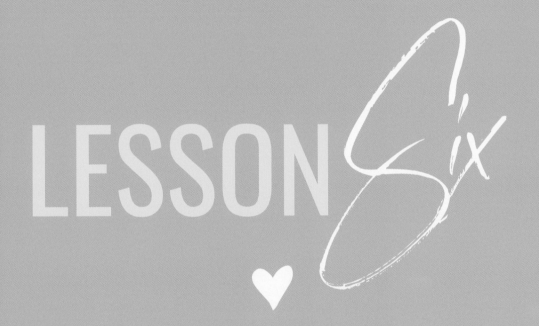

Your past does not equal
your future, unless you
decide to keep living there

WE

grow

THROUGH WHAT
WE GO THROUGH

I don't know anyone who hasn't had a 'tough' past. Shitty things happen to everyone and things don't always go to plan. I'm convinced that the stuff that happens to us really does happen for a reason, and even if, at the time, we don't quite understand why, one day we will.

It's so easy to be constantly viewing our past through the rear-vision mirror of our mind! We can find ourselves focusing on past events and replaying them over and over in our heads. Sitting with those unpleasant but strangely comfortable feelings associated with that event or person. Sinking into the sadness or grief that it left behind.

Not that you shouldn't be allowed to feel all of those feelings – because I genuinely believe you 100 per cent should. Feeling them all is very important, and we'll dive into why this is so important in the final chapter of this book.

For now, let me just say that there is no possible way to create an incredible future that is going to deliver you happiness, growth and great memories if you keep turning back to focus on the past.

Katie Dean, one of my life coaches and now also a friend, once said to me:

'If you are feeling depressed, you're living in the past – and if you are feeling anxious, you're living in the future.'

Are you drowning out the amazing moments happening to you right now, because you are ignoring the present moment and are stuck living in the past?

I believe that the best way to be happy is to be in the present and in the now.

Let go of what has happened, because there is nothing you can do about it now. And please stop worrying and wasting energy on the 'what ifs' of the future, because none of us knows what is coming.

At every opportunity, for so many years, my mind loved jumping back into the past. Examining what happened to me in my childhood was a particularly popular destination to revisit. I spent a lot of time stuck in a very negative headspace that was all about looking backward, not forward. I would get so envious of my friends, who I saw as being lucky because they hadn't gone through the same kind of hardships as I had. I would be miserable and feel so sorry for myself, instead of waking up with gratitude that I'm not only alive, but that I have choices, that I'm the author of my own story and I can change the chapters to suit the way I want my life to be. But that required me to stop living in the past.

Comparing your life to someone else's is just downright unhealthy and pointless. The whole comparison thing needs to stop. It never achieves anything, except to make us all feel terrible, that we aren't enough or don't have enough – which instantly positions us as victims.

Don't we all want life to be more enjoyable, less stressful, more exciting?

Letting go of the past is the best gift we can give to ourselves – the choice to do so is entirely up to us.

It takes time and effort to erase this very familiar pattern of behaviour. When I catch myself falling back into that mindset of dwelling in the past, I ask myself, 'What exactly will it achieve if I go back into what's happened?', OR, 'If this keeps popping into my mind often, then maybe it's not something that has healed for me, and I should be leaning into it rather than trying to ignore it?'

Although you might think the quick and easy way to avoid the pain is by ignoring these feelings, I really don't recommend it. We might be able to suppress the pain on the surface, but our subconscious will remind us we haven't healed. It will continue to cause us pain in some way or other until we face it head-on and work through it.

We grow through what we go through – and part of the healing process is to work through all of the feelings, stories and attachments that we have buried in our past. So many of us have struggled through rough patches in our lives, and we really need to learn to embrace it all, as all of our experiences have shaped the person we have become.

Our past does not equal our future. And who you were last year, or three, five or fifteen years ago, is not who you are today!

How frigging exciting is it that we have choice, freedom and some control over what we do with the next chapter of our lives? Always remember that you decide what happens next … so let's stop dwelling in the past and start getting excited for what's to come!

REMEMBER:

♥ Things change.

♥ People change.

♥ We change.

♥ Situations change.

♥ Circumstances change.

♥ What we need and value can change.

♥ Our lives can and will continue to change – every single day, every single season, and every single year.

WRITE DOWN
5 NOT-SO-GREAT
THINGS THAT HAVE
HAPPENED IN YOUR PAST

Then write down the positive
things that have resulted from
those negative experiences

1

2

3

4

5

Smoothies

Each recipe makes 1 serve. Add all the ingredients to a high-speed blender and whiz together until smooth

Peanut butter banana smoothie

1 cup milk of your choice (I love almond milk)

1 frozen banana, peeled and roughly chopped

4 tablespoons rolled oats

1 scoop vanilla protein powder

1 tablespoon natural peanut butter

1 cauliflower floret (don't worry, you can't taste this!)

Caramel almond smoothie

1 cup milk of your choice

2 tablespoons almond butter

1 scoop caramel coffee creamer (I love the BeforeYouSpeak brand)

1 scoop Happy Way salted caramel whey protein powder

a pinch of Himalayan salt

ice cubes

optional: 1 pitted date

optional: add 1 tablespoon Morlife's Caramel Almond Dough Clean Treats

Espresso açaí bowl

1 ½ large (150 g) frozen bananas, peeled and chopped

½ avocado

1 scoop vanilla protein powder

1 sachet (100 g) frozen açaí

1 sachet mocha coffee (I use Glow Mocha, by BeforeYouSpeak)

1 teaspoon cacao powder

a splash of coconut water or almond milk

optional: ½ zucchini, roughly chopped

Dragonfruit smoothie bowl

1 cup frozen strawberries

1 cup dragonfruit chunks

1 scoop vanilla protein

½ zucchini, roughly chopped

1 teaspoon açaí powder

a splash of almond milk

Choc oats breakfast smoothie

1 cup milk of your choice

½ cup rolled oats

1 tablespoon rice malt syrup or natural maple syrup

1 scoop chocolate protein powder (I love Triple Choc Fudge by Happy Way)

1 teaspoon cacao powder

Get your greens mango smoothie

1 cup almond milk

¼ avocado

½ zucchini, roughly chopped

100 g baby spinach leaves

100 g frozen mango chunks

1 scoop vanilla protein powder

Vanilla cinnamon smoothie

---

1 cup almond milk

⅓ cup rolled oats, or 1 frozen banana, peeled and roughly chopped

1 scoop vanilla protein powder

2 tablespoons natural maple syrup

2 tablespoons almond meal

1 teaspoon ground cinnamon

1 small handful ice

optional: blend in 1 teaspoon cacao nibs, to make it choc chip!

Blueberry choc coconut smoothie

---

1 cup coconut milk

100 g frozen blueberries

¼ avocado

1 scoop chocolate protein powder

1 teaspoon cacao powder

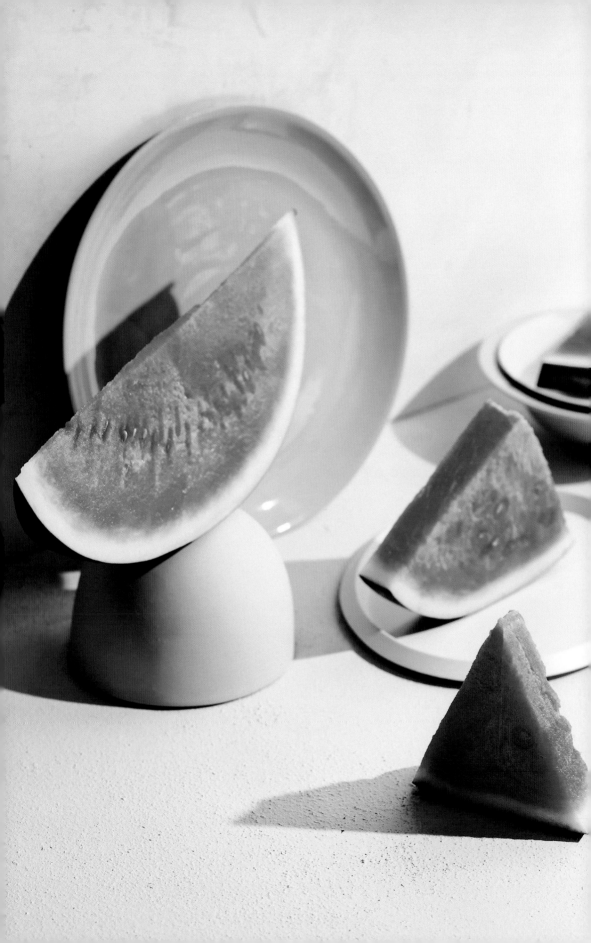

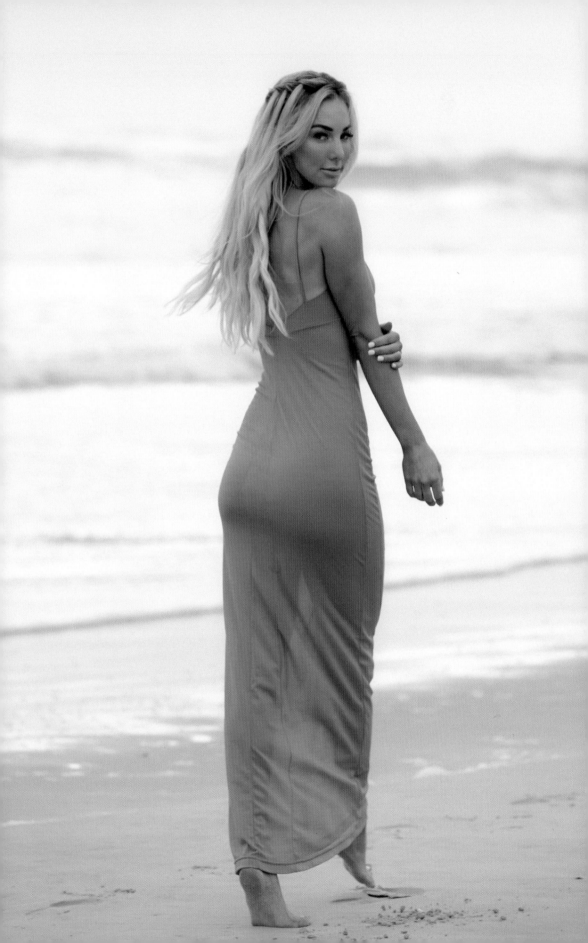

LESSON Seven

♥

Asking for help is not a
sign of weakness

Lean in

TO IT
DON'T RUN
FROM IT

Warning! In this chapter I'm going to get incredibly raw and real with you. Very few people know this story, as I've never before shared the extent of the dark times I went through a few years ago.

This story isn't something that's easy for me to share, and I did think very seriously before including it in this book. My decision to write about it stems from truly believing that someone reading this book needs to hear this.

If I can help even just ONE person who is going through something very tough in their lives or is feeling as low as I felt, then sharing this experience has been the right thing to do.

Like many of you, I've been through a lot in my life. Living my life so openly online over the last decade, and seeing my audience grow so much, has meant millions of people know me and follow my day-to-day life.

I am so very grateful to have a voice on such a powerful platform. So I am always trying to use that voice as an opportunity to help inspire and motivate others. That's the key reason I share so much of my own experiences and lessons online.

MY JOURNEY INTO DARKNESS

I have such gratitude for this life path I'm on and it's something I never take for granted – but there is also a darker side to being online.

Some of you may be familiar with this other, darker side. In fact, you might be experiencing it yourself or at least know someone who has been bullied online.

Being bullied is not new to me. Just like some of you reading this, I was bullied at high school. I didn't ever really feel like I belonged and couldn't find a way to fit in. It made me feel isolated, unloved and constantly judged. I felt criticised for, well, just being me. That's where my journey and lesson started.

As a teen, I definitely didn't know how to navigate through the difficult aspects of my life. I was dealing with bullying, self-doubt, self-sabotage and a crippling lack of self-belief.

I carried those wounds through to the next chapter of my life because I lacked the right guidance or knowledge to deal with them at the time.

These same behaviours, feelings and lessons would show up again many years later, but this time I wasn't being bullied in real life – the bullying was now online.

Yes, I do absolutely understand that by putting your life online, you have to accept and be okay with some people not liking you and with people judging you or just not agreeing with your point of view. Of course people are also going to have their opinion on pretty much everything you do, wear, eat and say. I totally get ALL of that.

I also thought I was pretty strong, and could handle quite a lot. But boy was I wrong!

HOW THE HATE BEGAN

A couple of years ago, a small group of girls decided they didn't like me, so they started a Facebook forum page where they could all gossip online about my life and everything I did. They loved to discuss my friends, my family, my son and my business ventures.

What started off as a small and petty gossip group soon exploded into much, much more. Their few hundred followers grew to be thousands and thousands.

A core group of five women in the group had created a roster for themselves, so they could watch ALL of my Snapchats and Instagram stories at all times. Their plan was to target me 24 hours a day. They would race to screenshot my posts and upload them to their forum so they could then make fun of me, tease me and create endless awful memes about me. They also encouraged their following to go onto all of my social media platforms and post negative comments on pretty much everything I posted about.

Some news media also started following the hate forum, trawling through the commentary searching for potential 'clickbait' headlines. Fuelling the hate frenzy, the forum followers would flock to the negative media stories and post the most awful and often unrelated things in the comments section about my son or my husband, the business – everything and anything!

This started an ongoing and what felt like a never-ending vicious cycle of constant negative press and headlines about whatever was going in my life – whether it was true or not.

Thousands of online trolls and the media were just bombarding me – with no let-up. This wasn't for just a couple of days or even a few months. This went on and on, for over a year. As each month passed, it all became harder and harder for me to live with.

It took me back to those feelings at high school, but in an amplified and much more public way. Once again, it felt like I had no voice in conversations that were ALL about me.

I felt I couldn't breathe.

I felt I couldn't be myself.

I felt like no matter what I did or where I went, they were watching – ready to pounce.

I felt like I was drowning, that this was now my life and I had NO CHOICE but to accept it.

THEN THE HATE MOVED TO REAL LIFE

It moved beyond the online, to something even more real and threatening.

When I was out in public, strangers would follow me and stalk me. They would take photos of me without my permission and then post them in the hate forum. I would have food thrown at me, I was pushed and shoved in shopping centres. There would be unknown knocks on my front door. One day, someone found my home address and posted it on the forum – which triggered a barrage of threats in my inbox from women letting me know they knew where I lived and that they were coming for me!

One time when Steve was away, I mentioned on my Snapchat how much I hated being home alone. Almost immediately, that post was uploaded on the forum.

Suddenly my phone started to blow up from hundreds of people messaging to warn me they were coming because they knew I was home alone.

I no longer felt SAFE.

Yes, I knew most of these were just empty threats – but I was still scared. At the time, I was a mum with a two-year-old child and I really didn't know what someone might be capable of doing.

As with most experiences in life, it can be hard to understand how something feels until you've been through the same thing yourself.

It does feel really lonely when you think no one else truly understands what you're going through.

It was pretty clear to those around me that I was in pain and not myself, and I do genuinely want to acknowledge how lucky I was to have such a supportive husband, family and circle of friends. Even some beautiful human beings online made sure to show me their love and support.

But it didn't change how I felt. I saw myself as a burden to everyone. I was always sad and not a great energy to be around. I found myself starting to withdraw from my loved ones. In my mind, I thought I was doing them a favour – but all it did was make me feel more alone.

So what did I do?

For way too long I felt I needed to just cope with it all myself, and get through it alone. Because I believed no one really understood what I was going through and I felt like a burden to everyone, I decided I'd try dealing with it on my own.

Simple fact is – I couldn't!

THE LOWEST OF THE LOWS

Instead, I hit a massive low. I didn't want to get out of bed for days. I could clearly see the pain it was causing to everyone around me, but I felt somehow paralysed and just couldn't think or see clearly enough to find a way out of it all. I felt like I'd lost myself and even though I didn't want to continue living like this, I didn't know how to make the haters stop or the headlines stop.

If I ever showed any sign of vulnerability online, or that I was struggling mentally or emotionally, it would create a frenzy on the forum. The haters loved it, they fed off it, it made them excited. It was as if they had won, or they thought I deserved to be this unhappy. I still can't understand how any human can actually enjoy seeing someone feel so low.

It reached a point where I didn't feel safe sharing my experiences or pain or admitting I was in a place I didn't think I could get out of – or even knew how to get out of if I wanted to try.

It was all so painful and horrible emotionally that I just wanted it to end.

I believed the only way to stop the pain and fear and no longer be a burden to my friends and family was for me to end my life. When you feel there are no other options – that's when the notion of ending your life comes into play. But I promise you there is always someone to talk to, to help you, to reach out to. No matter what position you feel you are in, you are not facing this alone. I promise you, you're not. That was actually such a beautiful thing for me to experience when I felt so alone – to step up and reach out and to see and feel the incredible support that was there. It just took me being brave and saying, 'Hey, I need some help.'

I just couldn't continue to live like that. Waking up in fear and hating my life. I was unable to focus on the positives or enjoy my day-to-day life. The online hate consumed me, and what I feel most sad about is how much my son Taj would have been feeling my sadness.

Once I hit this point, Steve knew it was time to get help – immediately.

REACHING OUT FOR HELP

Steve had recently taken a weekend course with life coaches Alexi Panos and Preston Smiles. He was blown away by their attitude to life, the way they view the world and how they work through challenges and emotions. Steve believed they were the ideal people to help get me out of the emotional hole that was threatening to drown me and my spirit for life.

Since they were based in Los Angeles, my first session with them was via Skype. I bravely faced them on screen and worked hard at pretending to be okay. Barely two minutes later, I had collapsed to the ground in tears, sobbing. I couldn't hold back. I told them I couldn't go on and wanted to end my life.

I begged them to help me because I loved my son, my husband and my family too much to leave them. I knew deep down that ending my life wasn't an option, but the place I was living in emotionally needed to change – and fast.

*Whatever they said in that moment is a blur to me
– but whatever they said gave me hope,
strength and a new focus.*

To be brutally honest, when they sent through their online coaching fees I almost fell off my chair! It made me even more stressed, and I said, 'Steve, I'm not doing this – we just can't afford it.'

That same day, Steve paid in advance for six months of coaching for me. His response was, 'We will always find a way, and this isn't a should we – it's an absolute must. There is nothing more important than your mental wellbeing and we will do whatever it takes to help you.' (Thanks Steve… I have no idea what would have happened to me without you!)

THE DARKNESS BEGINS TO FADE

I swayed between real excitement and pure fear of the deep work I was about to dive into. I trusted that this new focus, support and help I was going to receive would be life-changing. I felt like this was a lifeline for me. It simply had to be!

Meanwhile, the online hate did not stop. It did not slow down and it did not get easier. But something else did change…

I became stronger. I learned more about why the haters were hating. I also learned new tools to help me manage my own emotions and triggers. A lot of those feelings I'd experienced in high school were showing up again, but amplified tenfold.

Throughout my life, I've made a big effort to educate myself and absorb as much information as I can, from everywhere I can. I've done Tony Robbins courses, hired coaches, learned from the wisdom and smarts of my amazing husband, read lots of self-help books and listened to plenty of great podcasts. The one critical thing for me, and the biggest lesson and message that I want to get across right now is…

A lesson is repeated until it is learned.

SOMETIMES PEOPLE ARE MEAN

During each session with my coaches, I would normally vent whatever I was feeling – things I had heard, felt or sat with, but couldn't move through.

Obviously, there were a lot of tears and a lot of time spent being uncomfortable, but at the end of each session my coaches reminded me to change my focus and my meaning, and to find the lessons and gifts: that something that helps make you stronger or that helps you help others or that you can be proud you got through.

No matter what, coaches or not, we will all experience hard times and challenges, but if we can change our meaning and focus it, this can change not only our mindsets, but help us build resilience and the confidence to believe in ourselves and our purpose.

My coaches also reminded me that, more often than not, most of the things others would say about me had less to do with ME, and much more to do with THEM. I was like a mirror for them, so that anything THEY were saying I was, or was doing, was actually about who THEY were or what THEY were doing. However, as they didn't understand how to process this themselves, they would instead project it onto me as a coping mechanism.

Understanding that really helped turn me around from feeling like the victim and made me much more compassionate towards them.

The saying 'hurt people hurt people' really resonated with me. When someone is truly happy within themselves, they won't put others down – so when someone is bullying online, you just never know what has happened to them to make them act in that way.

Now, I'm not saying it's okay for them to be a bully, but when you can try to come from a place of understanding, you'll have more compassion and be less likely to react back at them and add more fuel to the fire.

MY TOP SIX BOOKS

Becoming Brave
Katie Dean

The Subtle Art Of Not Giving A F*ck
Mark Manson

Rising Strong
Brené Brown

Unshakeable
Tony Robbins

Awaken The Giant Within
Tony Robbins

The Power Of Now
Eckhart Tolle

I do believe that life or the Universe does sometimes whisper us a message in the form of an experience, some pain or a challenge. If we choose to ignore it, the message is likely to show up again – but if we learn from it, then it's likely to resolve and fade. Keep ignoring the whisper and the Universe will try harder to capture your attention and will deliver that lesson to you again and again, but in louder, more insistent and more demanding ways.

The more you ignore it, the more you will be forced to repeat that lesson, until you are finally forced to take action and work through it.

Please don't let it get to breaking point before you listen. Instead, listen carefully to the soft whispers that present themselves as small challenges, and choose to learn and embrace the opportunity to grow. Trust me: if you don't, that lesson will keep hitting you harder and harder until you don't have any choice but to act.

This is definitely something that's not easy for us to hear, and some-times I still feel myself slipping into that 'I was a victim of online harassment and bullying' mindset. But I now understand that this was my lesson and I appreciate that it happened to serve a purpose.

ALL OF US want to feel validated. We all want to be consoled and told it's not fair. Well, maybe for a short moment it's okay for us to indulge in a little 'pity party' – and I do sometimes allow myself to feel and sit in the emotions, because I believe that's a healthy thing to do. However, staying stuck in the victim mindset does not serve us. It does not help us at all. In fact, it just holds us back from growth and true happiness.

PERSPECTIVE IS EVERYTHING

I now realise my high school bullying experiences, along with the online hate I faced in more recent times, were lessons I needed to learn, primar-ily on how to self-love and self-soothe.

Through this incredibly difficult journey, I also learned one of my most valuable life lessons: the importance of compassion and understanding.

It's so true that 'hurt people hurt people'. When someone is directing their aggression, hate and anger towards another person, it's because they are usually carrying a lot of pain in their hearts, minds and bodies. It's so much easier to blame and point the finger than to take responsibility, be compassionate, be understanding and to always try to work from a standpoint of love.

Today, when I read something online that isn't nice, I try hard to remind myself that deep down that person doesn't want to be nasty. It's not really who they are at their core, and they don't really want to upset me, even though it may seem like they do. Being in that mindset, rather than the victim mindset, means I can respond and sometimes even help them in some way.

Yes, you read that right! It might mean helping them understand that their words might be a reflection of their own pain. It could be the ideal time to help them navigate through an old wound. Sometimes it's just as pure and simple as me giving love back to them.

It's never going to be enjoyable or necessarily get easier when people are nasty to you. I'm also not saying that I don't have days where I want to turn my phone off and pretend the nastiness isn't there.

What it has taught me is how important it is for me to stay grounded, stay strong with my energy and boundaries, and not be reactive. The more confident and proud I am of who I am as a person, the less it hurts. Today, I am much less concerned or worried about people who may say things about me that are not true. I don't take things personally because I know the truth.

I now choose to respond, rather than react.

I now choose new ways to deal with situations online and offline that are easier and nicer for myself and others. I've always tried to have pure intentions and want to continue to help others, as well as be a better person and an example for those around me.

Remember, if we are faced with hate either online or offline, we cannot control what another human does or says – but we can control how we respond to them.

I've learned that ignoring the feelings doesn't help. And that unleashing my own pain or anger back at them, or onto someone else, also doesn't help.

Another lesson I picked up on this journey is that we all make mistakes. We ALL do – and this is actually how we learn to do things better.

STOPPING THE CYCLE OF PAIN

My goal is to always come from a place of understanding. So if someone expresses anger, hate or anything unpleasant towards me, the first thing I do is check in with myself to see how it's feeling for me. If any pain or emotions do show up, then I lean into them to explore why. But I also like to check in with the other person to see if they are okay, and go deeper into what it is they are trying to say or express.

For me it's important that I try to hear them out, to see if there is actual constructive criticism there that I should think about taking on board, or if it is just someone being awful. It's easy to take things the wrong way online. We all know how easy it is to misread a text. Let's all learn the power of a love heart emoji. ;-)

I've also come to realise that if we want the world to change – to be kinder, to be nicer, to be more compassionate and understanding – then it all starts with YOU and ME.

Every day I try to be aware of my energy and my general state of being. There are definitely some days (for instance, that time of the month) that may not be the best day to address any kind of challenging issues. On those days, I'm better to just focus on my wellbeing and energy instead.

I wake up each day with the pure intention of sharing my life and experiences in the hope that it will help others. My mission is to help women connect and never feel alone. So now when someone says anything negative about me, it doesn't hurt as much or sting as much anymore.

COMING FULL CIRCLE

This rollercoaster ride of self-discovery has made me even more confident in myself and my mission. I know I'm on the right path to helping make the world a better place. My intentions and focus are on wanting to help and serve, but if someone doesn't understand that, see that or feel that, then it's not something I need to try to change or control.

The people who want and need my help know I'm here for them – and I'm not going anywhere.

Like I said, we're not always ready to hear a lesson from someone or maybe it's too triggering for us at this point in our lives. And that's okay, too. It's certainly not up to me to force that lesson or change my way of teaching to try to please everyone. My job is to be me, to be real, and to operate from a place of love.

When you know the truth, and your intentions and actions flow from love, it really doesn't matter what anyone else thinks or says about you.

Stand strong in who you are, your values, your beliefs, your purpose and your mission.

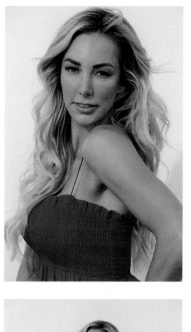
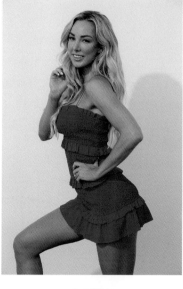
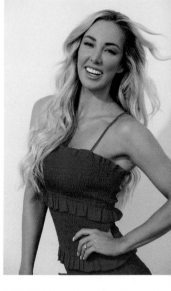
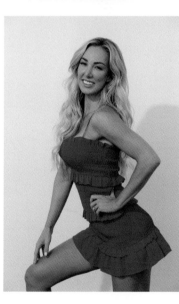
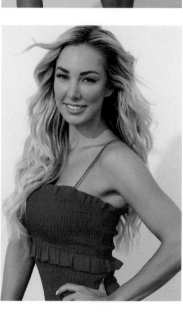
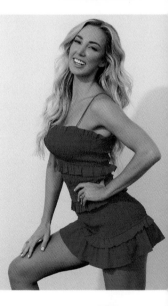
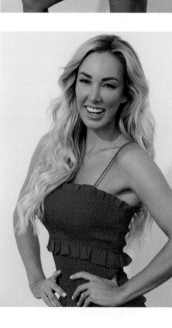
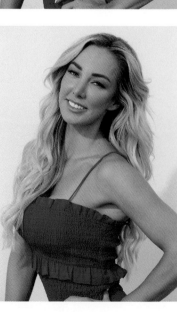
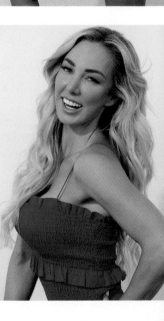

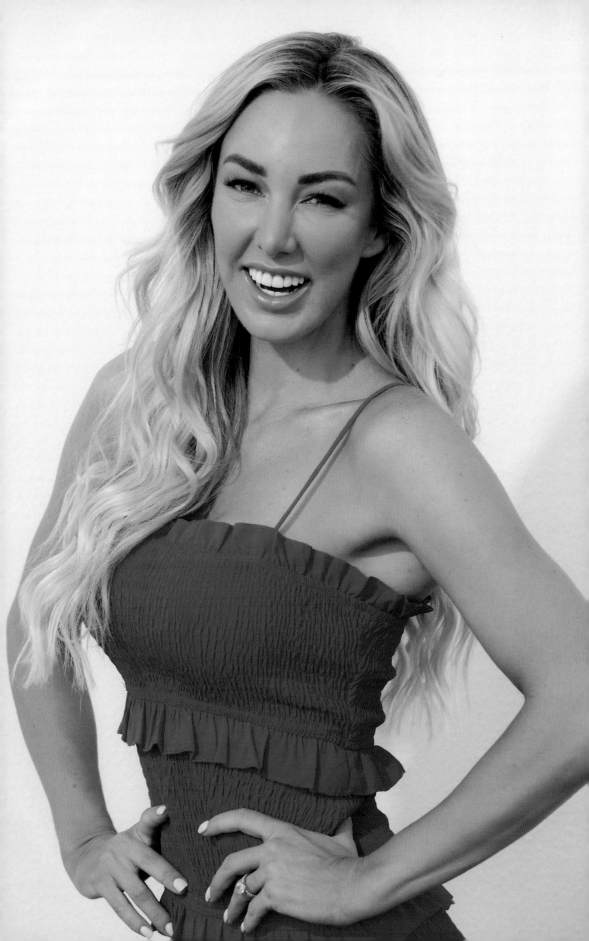

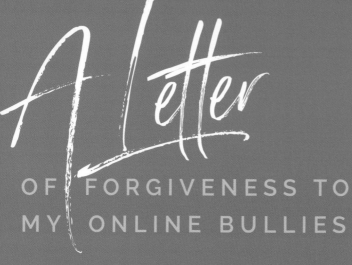

A Letter

OF FORGIVENESS TO
MY ONLINE BULLIES

I really do hope this letter finds you well.
I come from a place of peace and love. I don't hold any ill feelings towards you. How I felt then is very different to how I feel now…

I forgive you for hurting me.

I never spoke about the pain at the time, but it was unbelievably painful. It was so stressful that my body started to shut down. Everyone around me was affected and struggled seeing me this way. What you put me through was indescribable.

You broke me.
I thought I didn't want to be in this world anymore.

It was only after a long time that I was able to realise that the only way I could move on with my life and leave the past, pain and hurt behind was to forgive all those who had hurt me. Once I did that I found an inner peace and realisation of self-love. Looking back on it all now, I am truly grateful for the lessons.

- ♥ About compassion
- ♥ About hurt
- ♥ About pain
- ♥ About strength
- ♥ About ownership
- ♥ About self-love
- ♥ About letting go
- ♥ About freedom, because forgiveness sets us free.

I now know I can get through anything and I forgive you.

It's my hope that you can reflect back on this and have learned something too. I know that hurt people, hurt people. However, I believe we can all learn to respond a little more kindly.

I forgive you.

I saw you and heard you. I know you didn't mean it.

Sometimes I still catch myself drifting back to the pain I felt, but I've learned to let it go just as quickly as the fleeting memory. I no longer have the capacity, time or energy to feel that. I really hope you've learned that kindness is easy to give and can be spread anytime, anywhere.

I forgive myself.

Whenever I look at myself in the mirror I always want to be proud of who I am and how I interacted and treated people who came into my life. For me, true success isn't about how much money we have or what we own, but the real impact we have had on the people around us. We all make mistakes. I know I do, and I have, but I forgive myself for the mistakes I've made.

Growth is the key.

All of us have the capacity for growth and learning, as long as we can acknowledge our mistakes along the way. Say sorry not only to the other person, but also to yourself. If we all show up today being better people than we were yesterday, then we are doing well.

- ♥ Be kind
- ♥ Give love
- ♥ Show compassion
- ♥ Don't blame
- ♥ Ask for help.

Start each day with kind intentions to make a positive difference in the world. I really hope you've found love, happiness and peace in this world.

♥ *Ashy*

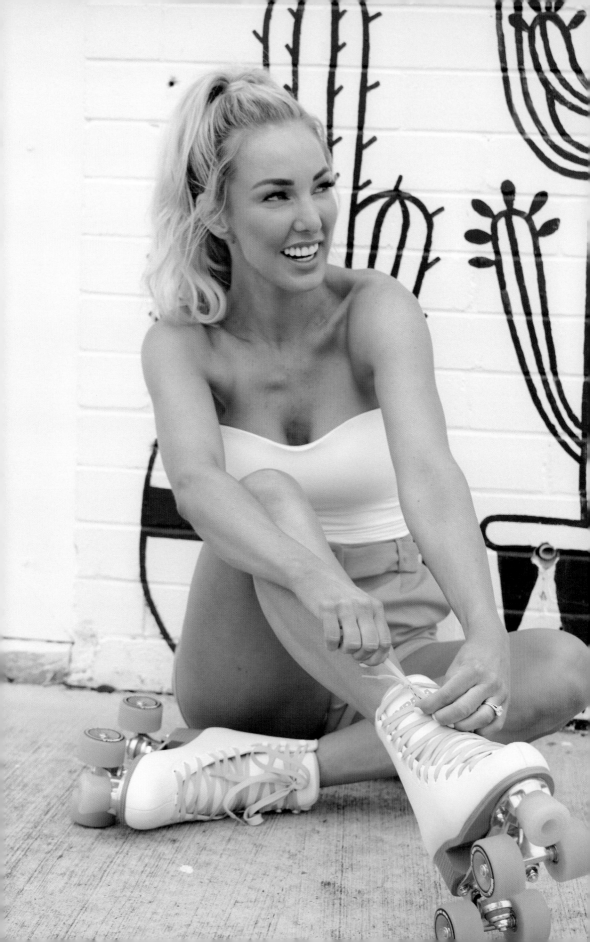

LESSON *Eight*

♥

Every moment is a chance
to learn and grow

TURN YOUR CAN'T
INTO CAN &
YOUR DREAMS

into plans

I can't wait to share this lesson with you – I'm sure it will be an actual game changer in your life! How would you like every single really challenging time in your life to be way less scary, less daunting and less exhausting? That would probably be a big YES PLEASE, right?

We all know that it is just not possible for us to control everything that happens to us, and that sometimes in life we are going to be dealt cards we never, ever expected. But instead of fearing or thinking the worst – let's try changing the meaning around it.

For example, let's assume the same thing happens to two different people: person A and person B. Let's look at their reactions…

Person A: 'Oh this sucks SO bad, this is shit, I can't change this. Oh well, I guess this is my shit life and it sucks for me. This shouldn't have happened, so what the hell am I going to do now? I just don't understand! Why did this happen to me?'

Person B: 'Eeeek! Okay, so this wasn't in the plan, so what's my next step? How can I change the path or direction of this challenge to serve me? What is this going to teach me? Okay, maybe I've got to learn this now, so then I'll be able to deal with future situations like this better. Awesome, yes this is unexpected and hard... but now it's actually forcing me to learn a new skill that will help me now and in the future – let's do this!'

See what I mean?

*Let's please all try to see everything as
an opportunity – not a burden.*

Let's also remember that life is happening FOR us, not TO us! (Thank you once again, Tony Robbins.)

*Life just doesn't need to be, or feel,
so hard and heavy.*

I always want life to feel lighter and be more enjoyable because, well, why not? Why does life have to be so hard and heavy all the time? If we can learn ways for it to be more enjoyable and easier, then great!

I remember being so, so scared to speak in front of the camera. (Yep, me – Snapchat queen and YouTube lover … and now camera lover!) I was absolutely terrified! It was the same when it came to public speaking; I dreaded getting on stage to speak at events. I would literally break out in a massive sweat all over my body and my heart would race like crazy. All I could feel was pure nerves and anxiety. But at the same time I felt such a strong pull to move through the experience so I could learn and get better at it – so I would deliberately do my best to lean in to the nerves. All because I was so driven by my passion to want to reach and connect with as many women as I could, beyond just through the screen. I really wanted to be amongst them in real life, to share that real, deep connection and help make a difference to their lives.

Before a recent speaking event in Sydney, I practised so much prior to the event and probably over-planned what I wanted to say. I just wanted to be prepared so that I could share as much as possible with the women who were making the effort to come along to hear me speak. But once I was up on stage and answering everyone's questions, I felt so comfortable and at home!

I felt SO ALIVE – like I was meant to be there.

Another time I was invited to speak on a panel at an event called 'SHE' which featured so many other incredible speakers, including Jules Sebastian, Lorna Jane Clarkson and Charli Kate Adams. As I walked towards the stage, ready to face 500 women, I could barely walk the short distance in my heels because I was so shaky from nerves. But as soon as I got up on stage, all I could see was everyone smiling and the excitement on their faces. I was blown away by that reaction – and so, so incredibly happy and grateful to be up there.

It showed me once again that every new opportunity, no matter how much it might scare us initially, is a chance to GROW and do MORE, to do better and to become better than who we were yesterday.

For me that's a daily goal: how can I improve myself daily?

Also, just a friendly community service reminder to you – and myself, too – that this new challenge that you are not looking forward to dealing with isn't going to disappear. I know it feels hard right now, but it's not going anywhere anytime soon, so you may as well try finding the positives so you can get through it – and maybe even enjoy it!

HOW TO MAKE CHALLENGES WORK FOR YOU!

I'm setting a challenge for you now. I want to make it your new mission to change the way you view and handle new and unexpected challenges.

From this moment on,

I want you to **catch yourself the moment you start using negative language, energy or meaning when you are faced with a challenge.**

Try to avoid creating more stress or making the challenge harder than it needs to be.

How can you swap how you see it to make it seem more exciting and more enjoyable?

How and where could this serve you in your future challenges?

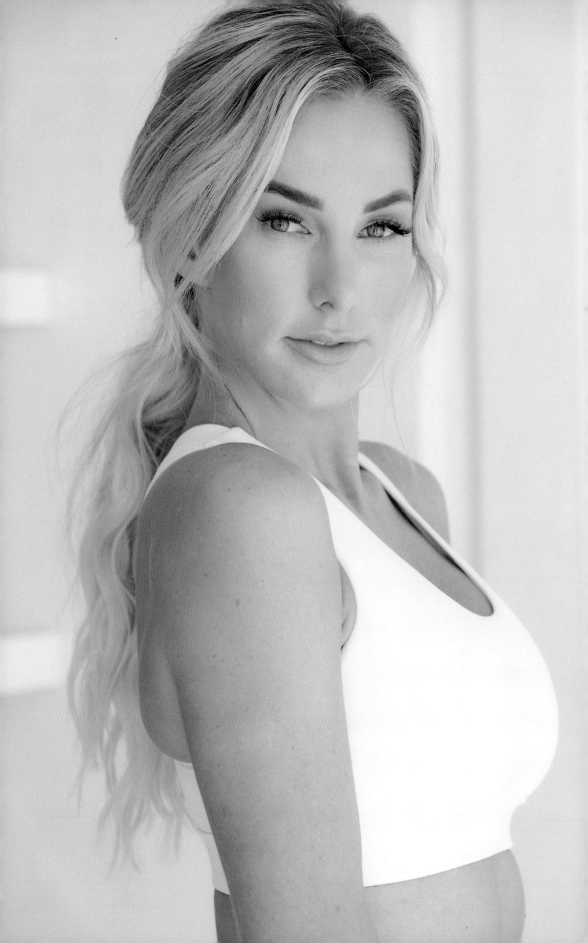

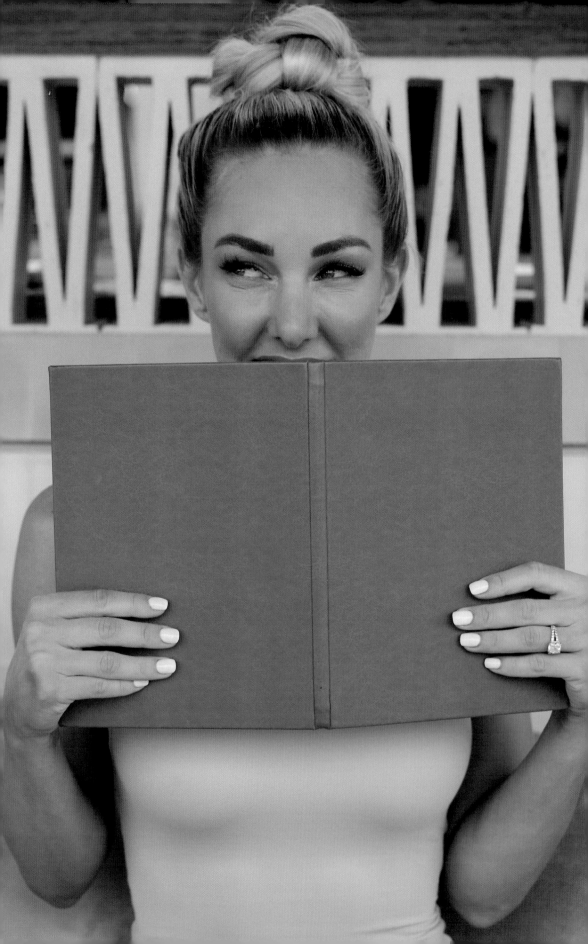

LESSON *Nine*

♥

Have faith and trust in the
universe. One choice can
change your life

EVERYTHING
HAPPENS AT
THE RIGHT TIME
FOR THE RIGHT
REASON

Trust

IN IT
FEEL IT &
EMBRACE IT

Sometimes I wish I had a crystal ball, and then other times – not so much. Yes, we can all go ahead and try to plan as much as we like, but I do believe the Universe has a plan for us, so that whatever decision we make IS the right choice.

But it's still really hard, when something happens in our life, to not allow ourselves to:

- ♥ fall into a 'poor me, why me' victim mindset
- ♥ point the finger of blame
- ♥ just feel sorry for ourselves that this is happening to us.

'Why me? What did I do to deserve this?' are probably thoughts that can easily pop up in your mind. Those questions would always flood my mind, too, until the day I finally kicked them to the kerb. That was the day I decided I was through with being the victim and feeling sorry for myself. I finally realised it wasn't serving me – it was only making me miserable!

Of course, none of us want crappy things to happen to us, but let's face the reality of life – unfortunately, it's not all rainbows and butterflies.

So let's drop the expectation that it should be simple and easy all the time. I've embraced the power of 'pressing pause' for a moment to take in a few big breaths and reset my mindset to one of trust and faith that everything happening right now is for a reason.

Yes, sometimes it sure can take a very long time before we know or understand why something happened. But we just need to trust that the reason will eventually be revealed.

Having trust can help to erase all the unnecessary anxiety and stress that we are probably feeling.

There have been a few times in my life where I've felt like my world was crumbling down around me. Looking back on those times, I can now see that in fact they were actually the BEST things to EVER happen to me! Let me share a few of these experiences with you, so you get the picture.

For starters, I'd be lying if I told you I didn't still wish that I had a dad.

Yes, I do still care! I would absolutely have loved to have had a dad who was there for me. Even on my wedding day, there was a moment where I felt such sadness about the fact that I didn't have a dad walking me down the aisle. As I always say, it's okay to feel whatever comes up.

Although I grew up without knowing my real father and went on to have a difficult relationship with my stepdad, I actually have them both to thank for so much. Both of those men are responsible for teaching me so many lessons, including some of the most important ones I needed to learn in order to become the person I am today.

TURNING IT AROUND

When I am going through difficult and challenging times and I just don't understand why they're happening, I ask myself the following questions:

♥ | What is this trying to teach me?

♥ | What is the positive in this?

♥ | What kind of meaning am I putting onto this situation? Positive or negative?

♥ | How much truth is there in this, and am I making it bigger than what it actually is because I'm scared or worried?

♥ | How can I move through this productively and not fall into my old patterns or habits of being a victim, thinking that 'Life is happening to me rather than for me'?

So many of the lessons they taught me, and so much of the growth I had to do as a result, are responsible for me being able to help all of you! They have also helped me to become the mother I am today, of which I'm extremely proud; it made me REALLY picky about my choice of life partner and, not surprisingly I chose incredibly well. All of this meant that I was able to find the very best father ever, Steve – and I now have a husband who loves me and treats me with so much respect. I feel blessed!

All of our past experiences, and the people in our lives or passing through, are here to help teach us and grow us in areas where we still need to do some learning.

My experiences with my dad and stepdad have also given me SO much gratitude that I have my mum. Some people take it for granted they have both a mum and a dad, and fully expect them to be around forever. But not having that positive male role model in my early years has made me hugely appreciative of my mum. Her strength, love and openness to grow and expand as an individual, a mother and now a grandmother has been phenomenal to watch.

If I hadn't experienced all that
I did as a child, I would not be who
I am today. I love who I am,
so the lessons were worth it.

The time I got fired from my sales assistant role in a clothing shop is another moment I want to share. How embarrassing, right? Well, yes, it definitely was, but it also came at a time when my car had been stolen and Mum and my two brothers had moved away. I just fell into a heap.

Mum and my stepdad were going through a relationship breakup. It was scary and traumatic for us all. My mum lost everything. Mum just wanted a new start. So she and my two brothers moved away. I made the decision to stay on the Gold Cast because by then I had met Steve and he made me feel so loved. It was hard not seeing my mum, but I knew that her being with my brothers was the best option.

I have two brothers. Matt is just 18 months older than me and we look very much alike. He's always been such a great protector of my mum and me. We share the same father – the one we never got to know. My youngest brother, Craig, is the son of my stepdad and he is the biggest sweetheart you'll ever met. I wish we could be closer but they still live interstate, so I don't get to see them often. They are such amazing uncles, and I know I could always call on them and they'd be there for me, come what may. I'm proud to have such beautiful people as my brothers! We have all stuck together through it all and we all have each other's backs, no matter what.

But back to that day I lost my job in the retail store... There I was with NO money, NO plan, NO direction and NO job.

The victim in me came out strong and loud – and the stories in my head played the same things over and over again and again...

'WHY ME?'

'Shit things always happen to ME!'

'I don't deserve this!'

Blah, blah, blah.

But ... if I didn't get fired that day, I would probably still be working in retail, folding clothes and vacuuming floors. Not saying there is anything wrong with that at all, and if that's your passion, then go for it. However, I always knew deep down that it was not what I was put on to this earth to do. I wanted to find a way to help people, but didn't know what that could look like or how to translate that into a career. Only when I became a personal trainer did I realise this new career was the gateway to achieving my dream to help others.

This was a dream I never, ever imagined would come true because of all the constant stories playing in my head, telling me that I was 'too dumb'. Had I not been fired, I would never have attempted to look into doing a personal training course. Honestly, I thought it would be a big waste of money, because of course I would fail.

SHOUT-OUT to the manager of the store I was working at – THANK YOU for firing me – or as she put it, 'letting me go'.

Being fired was the push I needed to go and study. When I got home from work that day, I bawled my eyes out, but Steve had already started getting things moving for me. Not only had he already organised where I was going to study, he'd also applied for government funding assistance, because of course I had zero money. This was exactly the kick along I needed to make change, to start living my passion and to start helping people.

Another experience I'd like to share with you is one I think we can all relate to – that very first break-up. Remember just how painful that first break-up was at the time? There are no walls or barriers and it's such a deep and all-consuming beautiful love. You truly believe that nothing can ever tear your bond apart…

You give so much to your first love because you're so fearless, having never been hurt in love before.

But then things start to fall apart, or maybe you simply grow up or grow apart, and then it ends.

Before meeting Steve, my absolutely incredible husband who lights me up in every way, I was so lucky to have had a reeeeally beautiful first boyfriend, Luke. He treated me like a queen, but as we both grew, much as I loved him and always knew I would, I realised I just wasn't 'in love' with him. I knew in my heart we needed to be on different journeys and find our own selves.

We had become very co-dependent on each other, which was not healthy, and we needed some space to really find out what it was that we truly wanted. I still never regret any moment we had together. He was my first love and one of my soulmates who helped to show me how I deserved to be treated.

Being so young, I had no idea how to end this relationship. I saw Luke as my best friend and had totally convinced myself that I would never, ever again find anyone as kind, sweet and caring – and cute! – as him. I didn't want to hurt him and seeing him in pain was my own worst nightmare. The break-up still haunts me to this day. Walking away from that relationship was an intense blur of immense pain, tears, anxiety and the deepest sadness of just missing each other.

If I'd had just had a little more trust in the Universe, I would have believed there would be another chapter for each of us that would give us someone who would make us feel completely loved and fulfilled.

I wish I had realised that, because it would have lessened the pain for us both. Yes, that first love break-up is such a hard experience we all go through. But if we learned to trust that everything happens at the right time, for the right reasons, then maybe the difficult experiences wouldn't be quite so scary or painful.

One more personal experience I'd like to share is one I think all women can also relate to. And I think you'll agree that this one is just as hard as losing a lover.

You all know how it is with best friends – we tell each other everything! We share all of our deepest, darkest secrets; we allow ourselves to be so open and vulnerable. There's so much trust and honesty exchanged, and some co-dependency as well. So when this one friendship ends, it really hurts deep.

I wear my heart on my sleeve, and I truly do love my friends just as much as my family. I've always valued friendship and always will. So, losing a friendship cuts me really deep. I have to admit that I even grieve when friendships change.

*Growing older, I've learned friendship cycles
are a very important part of our journey.
People come into our lives for a reason,
for a lesson or for a blessing.*

Some relationships and friendships are just not made to be a forever thing. They might not end because of a big blow-up; it can be that circumstances change, your life changes, your priorities shift, your connections, values and morals change. You simply might not have things in common anymore.

Even when you know all of this, it still hurts when it ends. I grieve through those changes and try hard to find the lessons. As I said earlier, I wish that in my past I'd had a little more trust that a friendship was ending for the right reasons. Trying to force something to continue that is no longer what it used to be is futile and just prolongs the pain.

I believe we have many soulmates – not just one! I remember a particularly close bestie who I lived with, trained with, worked with and played with – we were inseparable. We did everything together, and all we did was just laugh and have fun. This was a special friendship – we even had matching tattoos (although I've since had mine removed). One day, completely out of the blue, she packed up her stuff and messaged me to tell me she was off because she needed to start her life fresh. That's it – she was gone – and that was the end of our friendship. I had lost my best friend overnight.

Wow, that hit me like a ton of bricks. She had just moved away and didn't speak to me or any of our other friends. The end!

But no, not really. Just a few weeks later, Gretty, one of our mutual friends, needed a room – and, guess what, I now had a spare one! Gretty had done my challenges and I was her trainer, so it seemed like a fine idea. The rest is history. We've been besties for nearly a decade. In that time, we've worked together, started a business together, both had our beautiful babies, and I am so grateful to have her in my life every day!

That experience really helped me to learn to trust that everything happens for a reason. If that other friendship didn't end, then it's highly unlikely that I'd have such a close friendship and bond with Gretty. I love our friendship – it's a much more independent relationship, yet we're super-close. This is a much more mature friendship that I believe will last a lifetime.

When something falls apart, it's because it's creating the space for better or more aligned things – like the opportunity for new relationships to form and come together.

Believe that everything happens at the right time, for the right reasons. And, no, you may not find the gift or lessons or reasons straight away, but just sit back and trust that the Universe has your back and good things are coming. One day, you'll look back into the past and say, 'Ahhhhhh – that's why that happened! Thank goodness it did.'

Let's stop being afraid of what can go wrong and start being positive about what can actually go right!

Remember, one choice, one event, one happening
CAN change your life!

LIST THREE THINGS YOU'VE DONE, BUT NEVER BELIEVED YOU COULD

Then, next to each, write down the key reason
you were able to achieve this.

1

2

3

LIST THREE THINGS YOU DON'T BELIEVE YOU CAN DO

Then, next to each, write down what is holding
you back and how you can change that.

1

2

3

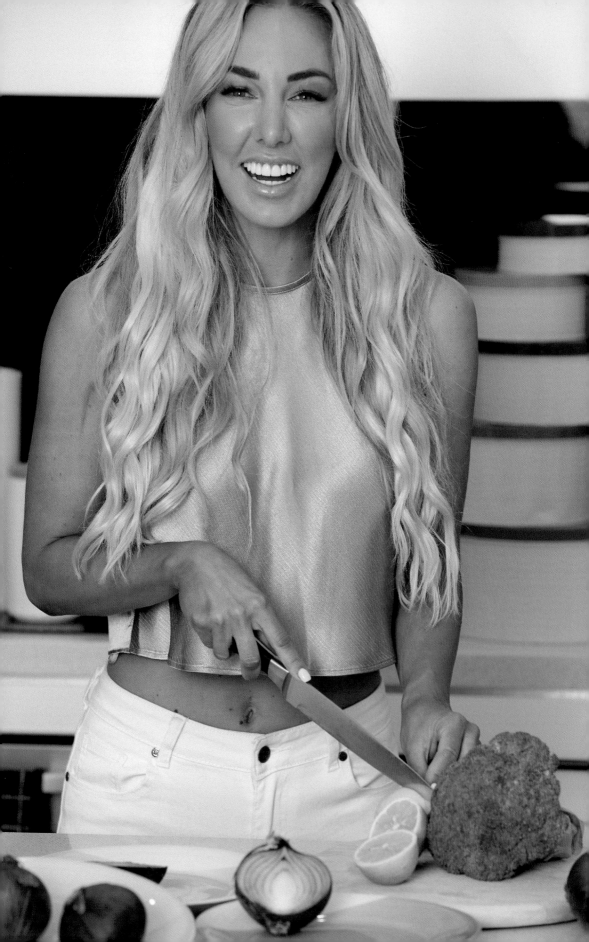

LESSON *Ten*

♥

Health always needs to be a priority

WE ARE A RESULT
OF OUR CONSTANT

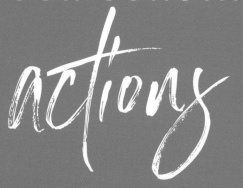

actions

When most people think of Ashy Bines, they probably think of 'that fitness girl'. My journey in the health and fitness industry first started when I was just 17 and got a job as a receptionist in a gym. I absolutely fell in love with the health and fitness world from that very moment. What I really loved was being part of something that was helping others to become fit, strong and healthy.

By the time I hit 20, I was a qualified personal trainer. Along the way, I became addicted to helping people transform their lives and lifestyles to be healthier. Being a part of their transformation journey, I saw them achieve so much, not only with their health, but in so many other areas of their lives. What I saw time and time again was that it all starts with a solid foundation of health, plus strength, inside and out – and I'm talking mentally, physically and emotionally.

I'm sitting here feeling pretty proud that I'm writing about how much I prioritise health on a daily basis, even during challenging times and when I'm travelling. But there have definitely been times when I've let things like work get in the way and I haven't made health my priority. That's when I can really notice just how much my general health affects the way I function. It makes such a big difference to my energy levels and mood – not to mention bloating. My skin health deteriorates and my digestion is impacted. Even my sleep suffers – I find I just don't sleep as soundly or as deeply.

All these side effects have a negative flow-on effect on my everyday life and even on how I interact with those around me, who I love so much. When I'm tired, grumpy, feel bloated, sick or even unconfident, it affects my energy, and everyone around me can sense that. It means I have less patience with my beautiful child and I definitely don't speak to my husband as nicely as I'd like to when I'm tired. I love my little family – so that's the last thing I want for them.

So this is a big wake-up call to remember that looking after your health is not just about looking great in a bikini or being shredded or really toned or not having cellulite. Our health impacts every single area of our lives, every single day. So I cannot stress enough the importance of making health your priority every single day.

No, it doesn't have to be super-overwhelming, and you don't have to make massive changes in your life. I would just like you to try to think about how much the little things you do every single day add up over the months, and over the years. Truth is – they add up to a lot!

Taking care of our bodies and nourishing our bodies isn't just about wanting to look a certain way. It's more about how it makes us feel and what it does for our mental wellbeing and energy, and ultimately our lives.

Your day-to-day actions, steps, routines and habits are key to who you will become. Remember, it all adds up!

Try thinking about it from this perspective: if you speak to yourself like crap, eat crap, drink crap and barely move – guess how you're going to feel? Pretty crappy, right?

Can you also guess what the results will be in your work, your relationships and how you feel about your life? Pretty crap, is the answer!

If you look after your body, feed your body nutrients, speak to yourself kindly, move your body, stay hydrated, stay connected emotionally

HEALTH ISN'T JUST ABOUT WHAT YOU EAT OR DRINK

To be truly healthy, we need a good balance of the following:

Good nutrition

Happiness

Family

Fitness/movement

Relationships

Energy

Feeling grounded

Mental wellbeing

Growth

Variety

Security

Safety

A sense of belonging

Love

with yourself and those around you and focus on living more intentionally – guess how you'll feel? Pretty damn amazing.

Only our consistent actions will give us the results we want. If you're consistently feeling crappy, low on energy, exhausted, grumpy and sick, then you need to look at your day-to-day actions and habits. Poor health is most likely why you are feeling this way.

Poor health = poor physical, mental & emotional state + poor energy

Choosing to be healthy doesn't have to be hard or unenjoyable. Many people might think that they have to stick to eating just lettuce or chicken and greens to be 'healthy', but that's just not true. My ongoing passion is to help women and their families find a new way to nourish their bodies that they can ALL really enjoy.

Let's remember that we can have a healthy lifestyle that is enjoyable and sustainable. No one wants to get back on that rollercoaster of yo-yo dieting and living, because that is no fun for anyone. So, finding food you enjoy and look forward to is important, and finding ways to make it as healthy as possible is the goal.

I love chicken parmigiana, but if I order it at a surf club it usually comes fried in breadcrumbs, in who knows what kind of oil. It gets covered in a sauce that includes unknown ingredients that are probably loaded with sugar. Then it is layered with three times the amount of cheese than I'd use at home. And let's not forget that massive side of hot chips… Yes, it's yummy, but do I feel good afterwards? Hell no!

But when I prepare it at home, which I do very often, it's a homemade chicken schnitzel, or a chicken breast sliced in half, with an organic no-sugar pasta sauce, one layer of lactose-free cheese (because I have trouble digesting dairy) and a generous side of veggies or salad. So my version is half the calories, but probably triple the amount of nutrients! Importantly, I'm not missing out on one of my fave meals. If I feel like having hot chips on the side, I'll chop up my own potatoes or sweet potatoes and oven-bake them – which are still so, so delicious, but way healthier. In fact, I actually prefer making my version now because I know it won't make me feel bloated and lethargic.

ASK YOURSELF
THESE QUESTIONS:

What kind of life do I want?

_____

_____

_____

Who do I want to be for those around me and what does that require?

_____

_____

_____

How can I be that person?

_____

_____

_____

How can I create that life?

_____

_____

_____

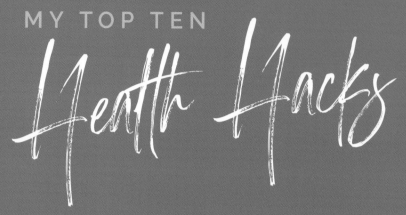

MY TOP TEN

Health Hacks

1. Start your day with water. Hydration always needs to be a top priority for overall health. If you're someone who forgets to drink water, set an alarm on your phone to remind you to hydrate. Keep a glass of water next to your bed, keep a bottle of water on your desk, buy a cute cup you love . . . whatever you need to do – because hydration is key!

2. Swap out all white bread, pasta and rice for brown or wholemeal versions. An easy swap that still tastes amazing but is much better for you health wise.

3. What is your food weakness? Find a healthier alternative. I love hot chips, so baking my own sweet potato fries is an equally delicious but much better option. I love chocolate, too – but now I make my own 'clean treats' that hit the spot every time.

4. Catching up with friends? Do some research to find healthy, yummy cafes in your local area, so you have no choice but to order a healthy meal instead of something deep fried!

5. Clean out your pantry and do a fresh food shop. I find it so motivating to look in my pantry and fridge when they're filled with colourful, fresh, healthy ingredients. It motivates me to want to cook, rather than order in.

6. Be prepared. If you're always on the go like I am, then make sure you have nutritious snacks in your bag, or prepare your meals the night before. Don't use time as an excuse for your choices; instead, make it a priority by making time.

7. Did you know it takes quite a few weeks to break a habit? Set your-self a goal to give up something that isn't serving your health. It might be takeaways or soft drinks, whatever that thing is for you. Walk away from it and I promise you'll feel better after 21 days without it! Not only will you see the difference in your body and feel good – the sense of achievement will motivate you to keep going.

8. Aim to do some type of movement every single day. If you've followed me on social media for a while, you'll understand how much my mind-set has changed when it comes to exercise. Back in the day, I used to put my body through what I'd call 'Smash and Bash'. Meaning I would overtrain and be so hard on myself, and feel so, so guilty if I wasn't at the gym six times a week training like a crazy person. Today, I move primarily for my mental health. Most days, it's simply a walk while either listening to a podcast or catching up with a friend, or maybe just listening to the sounds of the ocean while I'm gathering my thoughts for the day ahead. What an evolution – right? It's absolute bliss.

9. Listen to your body. Our body sends our mind so many messages – all day, every day. Often, a message just starts as a whisper, but it can get a lot louder if we ignore it. That initial whisper might escalate to a roar during those hard times in life when we are going through emotional or physical pain.

- ♥ If you have a headache, what is your body telling you? Not enough sleep? Not enough hydration? Too much stress?
- ♥ If you're feeling tight around your neck and throat, that restriction and tightness can signal to you that you're feeling shut down and unable to communicate.
- ♥ Check in with yourself often, every day, and ask yourself simple things like: Am I hungry? Am I thirsty? Why am I craving this? Is it because I didn't include enough nutrients or calories in my last meal? Am I depriving myself?

10. Try new recipes and foods. Add different herbs and spices to your meals and generally just have some fun getting creative in the kitchen. Once you've landed on a solid handful of recipes you love – such as the ones in this book, I hope! – then it really does make it so much easier to make quick, healthy meals on the go. Being more confident and prepared will make you far less likely to reach out for those unhealthy or fast-food options that don't serve your health, energy and moods, short term or long term.

THREE EASY WAYS TO SAY 'HI' TO HEALTHY HABITS

1 **Take a really good look at your morning routine.** How you start your day sets up your whole day. Start with a few deep breaths, hydrate with a glass of warm lemon water – and then go and MOVE. I'm not suggesting you go smash yourself in the gym for two hours. It can just be for 10 minutes, half an hour – however long you can manage. Just choose any form of movement that brings YOU energy and makes YOU feel good.

2 **Create a goal to introduce just three small new healthy habits to focus on for the next few weeks.** Trying to change too much too quickly can be overwhelming and can lead to giving up too soon, because it all feels too hard and stressful. For example, when I found out I was pregnant, the health of my baby and myself definitely became a priority, so I decided to commit to three healthy habits that I would stick to for the entire pregnancy, no matter what. The first one was to walk every single day. Number two was to drink a veggie juice every single day to ensure I was getting plenty of good nutrients, vitamins and minerals into my system. Habit number three was to drink 3 litres of water daily. Hydration is definitely something we all need to stay on top of, and when I was pregnant I knew I was responsible for someone else's health and wellbeing, too. Having those three simple habits to focus on really helped keep me on track. It wasn't too hard or too overwhelming ... and guess what? I stuck to all three – which made me feel so proud.

3 **Make sure you are actually enjoying your new change – especially when it comes to food and training.** If you are forcing yourself to eat something because you think it's 'clean' or 'healthy', but you actually dread eating it, then that is not going to work for you! Or if you start doing a form of exercise you hate, then I promise you won't last the distance.

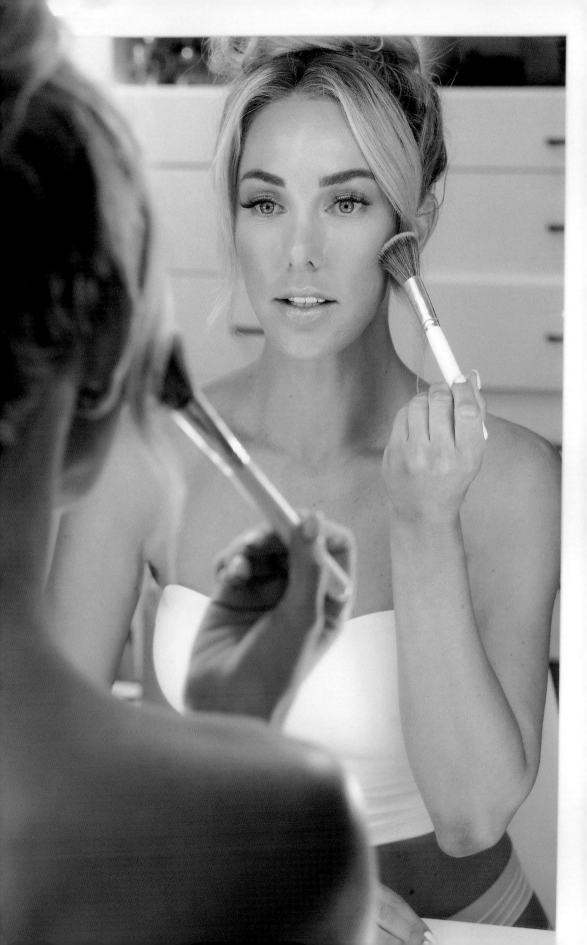

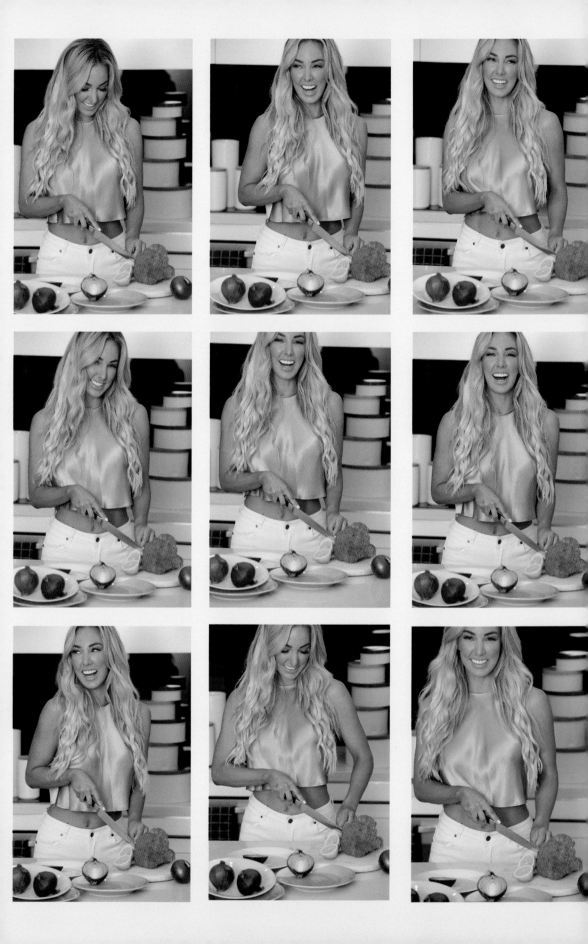

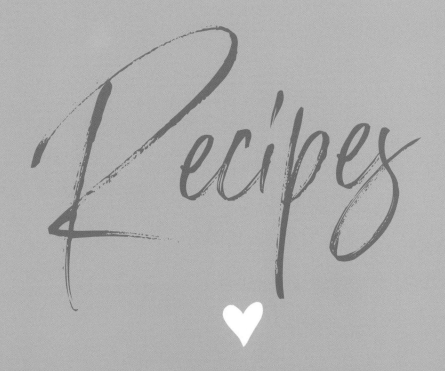

Recipes

♥

BREAKFASTS & LUNCHES

Here are some of my favourite fast,
simple and delicious everyday recipes.
Try them and feel great inside and out!

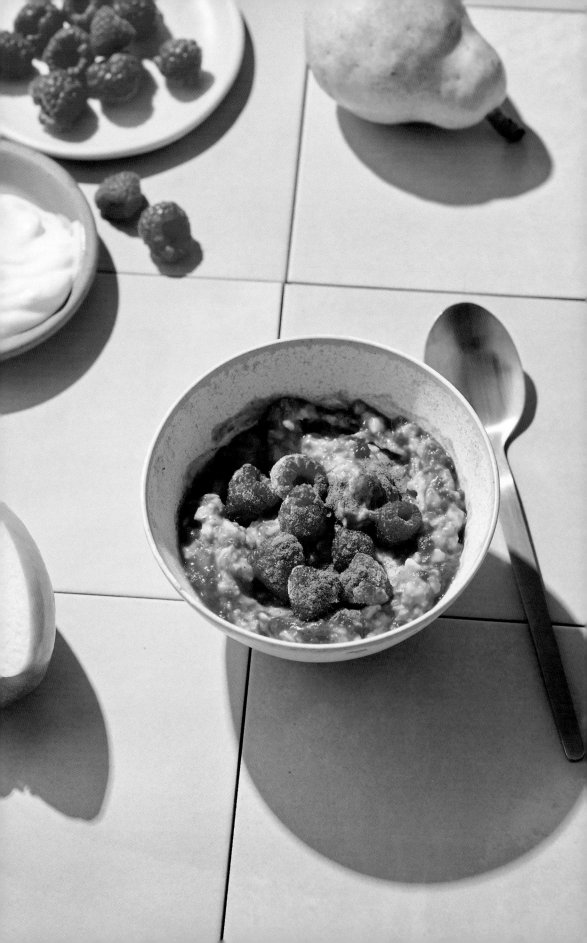

Raspberry cinnamon oats

Serves: 1–2 · Prep: 1 minute · Cook: 5 minutes

½ cup oats

1 handful frozen raspberries, plus extra to serve

3 heaped tablespoons coconut yoghurt

½ teaspoon ground cinnamon

Add the oats to a saucepan, cover with water and bring to a simmer.
As the mixture begins to bubble, start stirring to make a thick, creamy
oat mixture.

Stir in the raspberries and yoghurt.

Pour into a bowl, top with the extra raspberries and cinnamon and serve.

You can change the raspberries for any
other berry, or sliced apple or pear.

Spicy menemen

Serves: 1 • Prep: 5 minutes • Cook: 20 minutes

1 tablespoon olive oil

½ red onion, sliced

½ small red capsicum, diced

2 garlic cloves, sliced

2 small chillies, sliced

½ teaspoon smoked paprika

½ teaspoon curry powder

½ teaspoon ground cumin

200 g tinned tomatoes

Sea salt and freshly ground black pepper

2 eggs

Parsley, roughly chopped, to serve

Multigrain sourdough toast, to serve

Preheat the oven to 180°C.

Heat the olive oil in a small ovenproof frying pan over a medium–high heat. Add the onion, capsicum, garlic and chilli. Cook for 3–4 minutes, until softened. Stir in the paprika, curry powder and cumin and cook for a further minute, stirring occasionally.

Reduce the heat to low, add the tomatoes and season with sea salt and freshly ground black pepper. Simmer for 5 minutes, stirring occasionally.

Using a large spoon, make two wells in the tomato mixture for the eggs. Crack an egg into each well.

Cover the frying pan, place in the oven and cook for a further 10 minutes or until the eggs are cooked to your preference.

Sprinkle with parsley and serve with sourdough toast.

This creates a really spicy menemen. If you prefer a little less heat, reduce or omit the chilli.

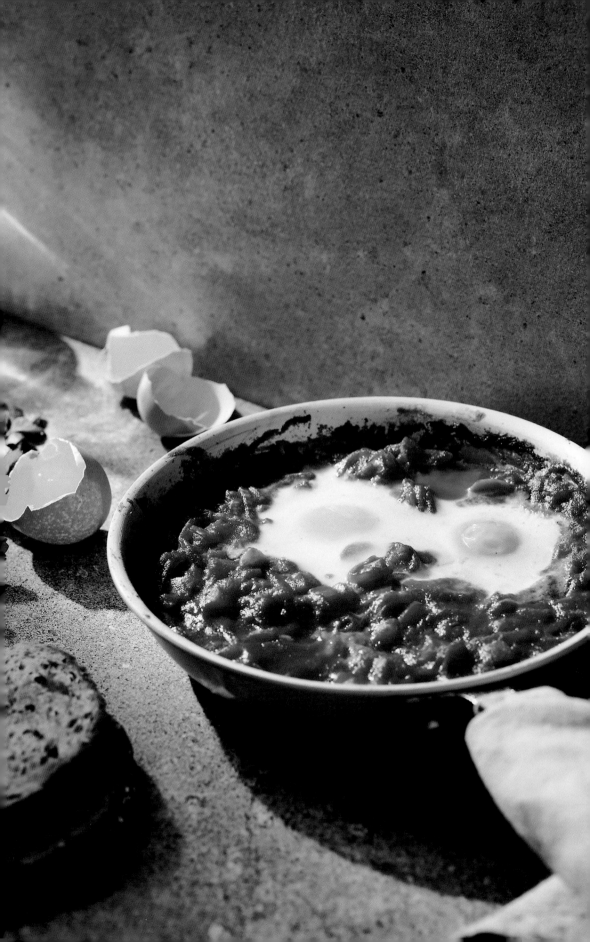

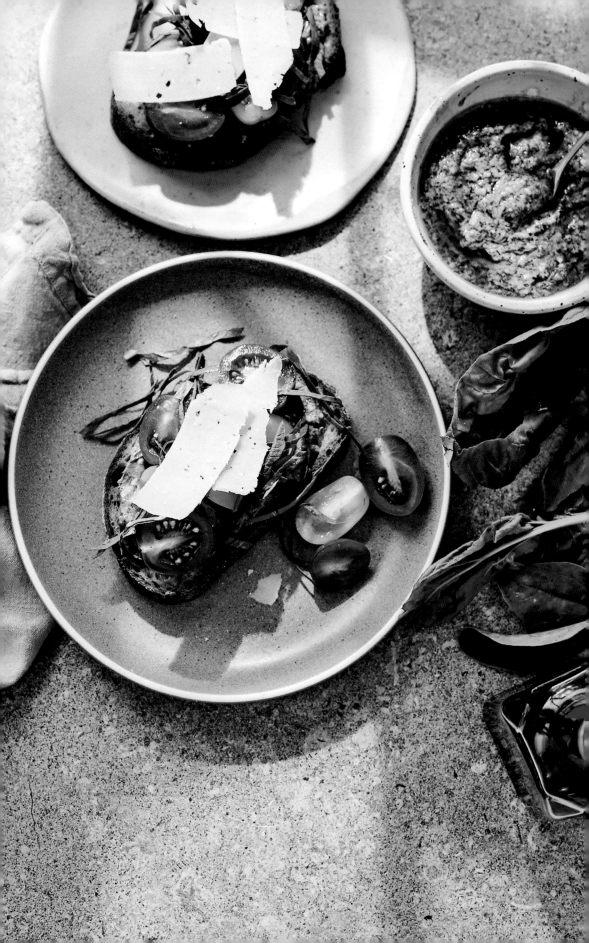

Pesto breakfast bruschetta

Serves: 1 • Prep: 2 minutes • Cook: 3 minutes

1–2 slices your choice of bread,
such as multigrain or sourdough

Basil pesto

Rocket or baby spinach leaves, finely chopped

Cherry tomatoes, halved

Parmesan, grated or thinly sliced

Balsamic glaze

Toast the bread, then smear with the basil pesto. Top with the rocket,
cherry tomatoes and then parmesan, drizzle with balsamic glaze
and enjoy!

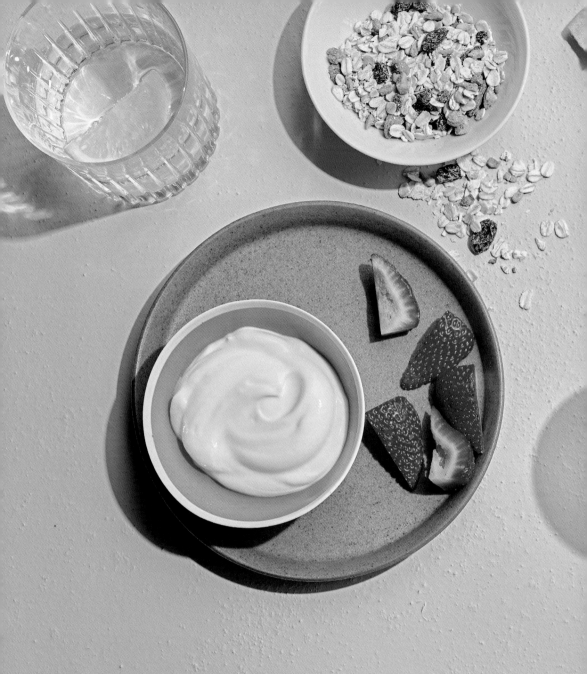

Fave sweet breakfast

Top right, recipe on page 145

Thick creamy açaí bowl

Bottom right, recipe on page 145

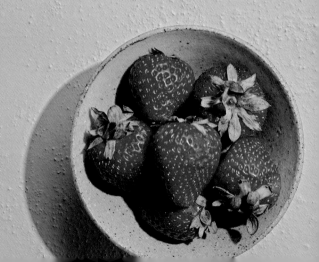

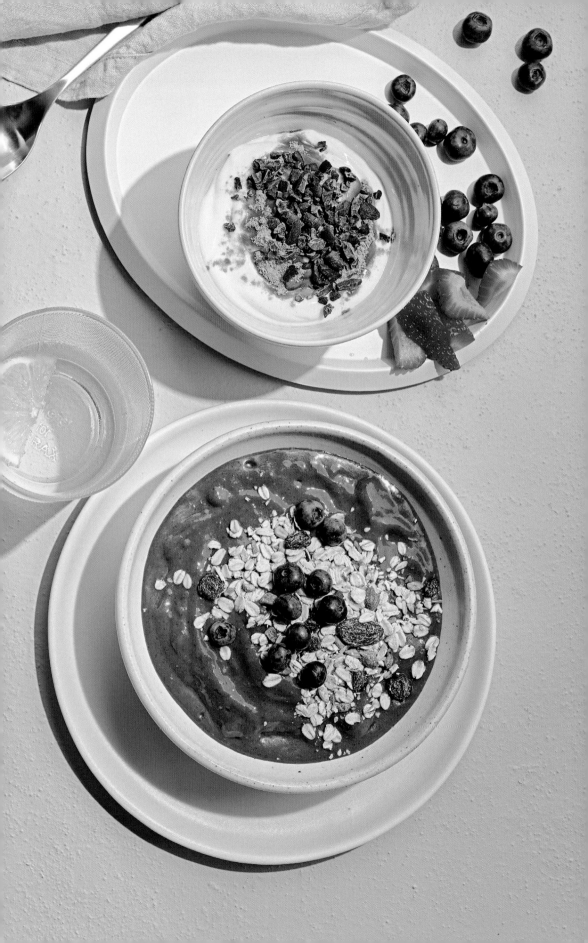

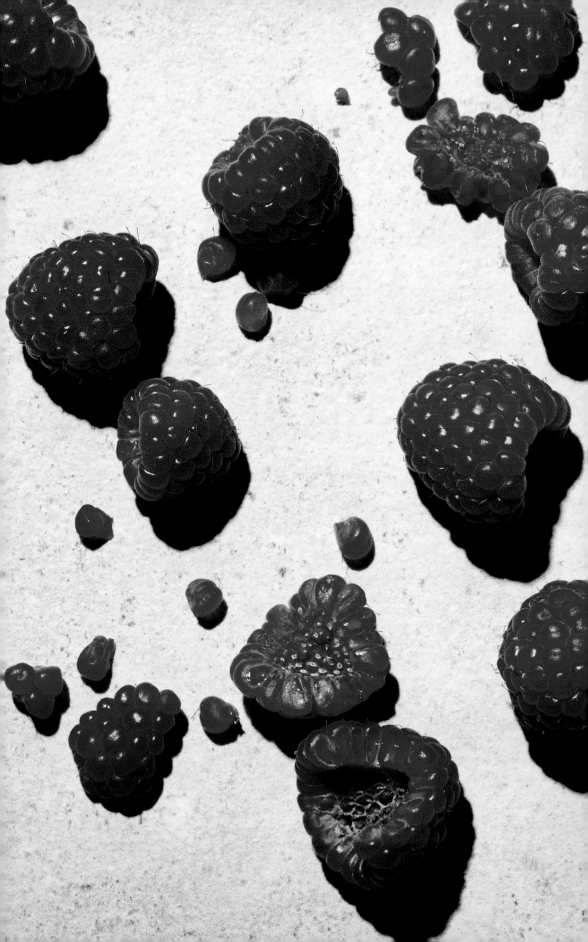

Fave sweet breakfast

Serves: 1 • Prep: 1 minutes

½ cup vanilla coconut yoghurt

1 scoop protein powder of your choice
(I love Happy Way Triple Choc Fudge)

1 tablespoon cacao nibs

Optional: strawberries or other berries of your choice

Mix all the ingredients together and serve with berries if you like!

Thick creamy açaí bowl

Serves: 1 • Prep: 2 minutes

2 frozen bananas (peeled and roughly chopped)

1 sachet (100 g) frozen açaí (I use Amazonia's Açaí Energy blend)

1 scoop protein powder of your choice (I love a chocolate hit and
a whey protein will make it even creamier)

⅓ cup almond milk

Add all the ingredients to a high-speed blender and whiz together
    until smooth.

Pour into a bowl and add toppings of your choice – I suggest strawberries,
    cacao nibs and a low-sugar muesli for texture and crunch!

Mum's gluten-free sweetcorn fritters

Makes: 10 fritters · Prep: 10 minutes · Cook: 15 minutes

grapeseed oil, for cooking

½ red or brown onion, finely chopped

1 cup gluten-free self-raising flour

2 eggs, at room temperature

½ teaspoon sea salt

½ teaspoon freshly ground black pepper

½ cup chilled soda water (the colder the better)

2 cups corn kernels (fresh, frozen or tinned)

Optional extras:

Coriander, parsley, mint or chives, chopped

½ cup bacon bits, cubed (fried with the onion)

⅓ cup feta, crumbled

Heat 2 teaspoons of oil in a frying pan. Soften the onion over a medium–low heat for about 5 minutes, until translucent but not browned. Set the onion aside in a small bowl.

In a large bowl, whisk the flour, eggs, salt, pepper and soda water into a smooth batter. Set aside to rest for 10 minutes.

Add the corn and onion (and any optional extras) to the batter and mix to combine.

In the same frying pan you used for the onion, heat enough oil for shallow-frying. Add 2 tablespoons of the fritter mixture and cook for about 2–3 minutes on each side, until golden brown. Repeat.

Serve immediately, while crispy on the outside and fluffy in the centre.

Mum loves to serve these with avocado and tomato chutney. No avocado for me! You can increase the quantity of corn kernels if you like your fritters loaded.

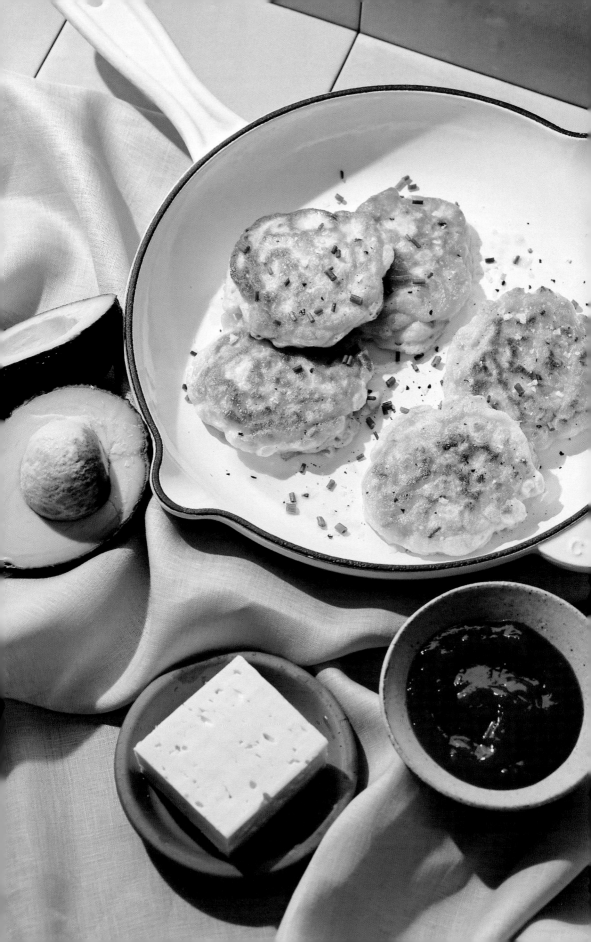

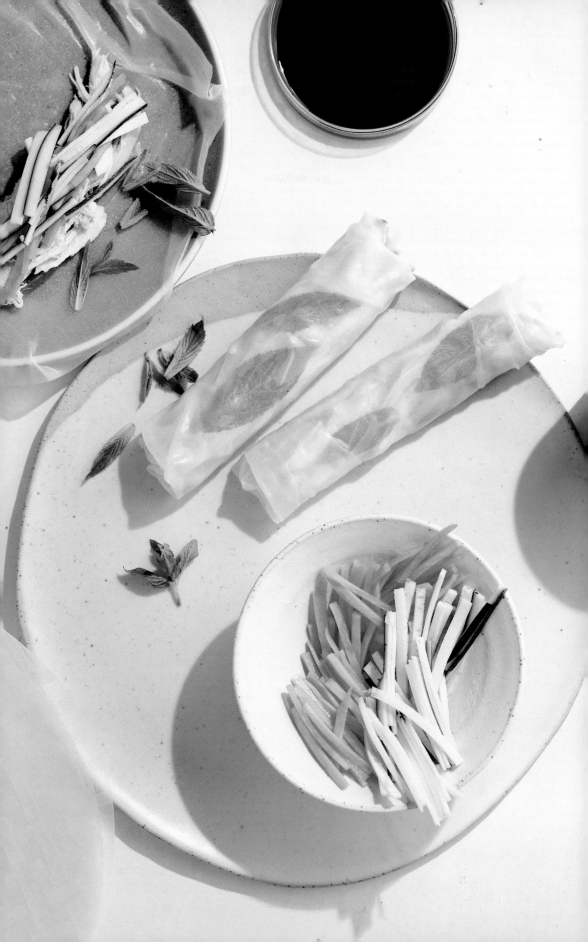

Chicken rice paper rolls

Serves: 1 · Prep: 5 minutes

2 tablespoons tamari

1 tablespoon olive oil

1 tablespoon coconut aminos

3 sheets rice paper

½ zucchini, cut into sticks

¼ carrot, cut into sticks

1 cooked chicken breast, shredded

Mint leaves

Make a dipping sauce by mixing the tamari, olive oil and coconut aminos in a small cup until combined.

Add hot water to a large heatproof bowl. Working with one sheet at a time, briefly soak the rice paper for about 10–15 seconds until softened and pliable (not too long or the sheets will tear).

Remove the rice paper sheet and place on a plate. Add one third of the zucchini, carrot and shredded chicken, top with mint leaves and roll up into a parcel. Repeat with the remaining ingredients.

Dunk the rolls in your dipping sauce and enjoy.

Swap in whatever salad or protein sources you prefer.
For a sweeter sauce, add 1 teaspoon rice malt syrup.

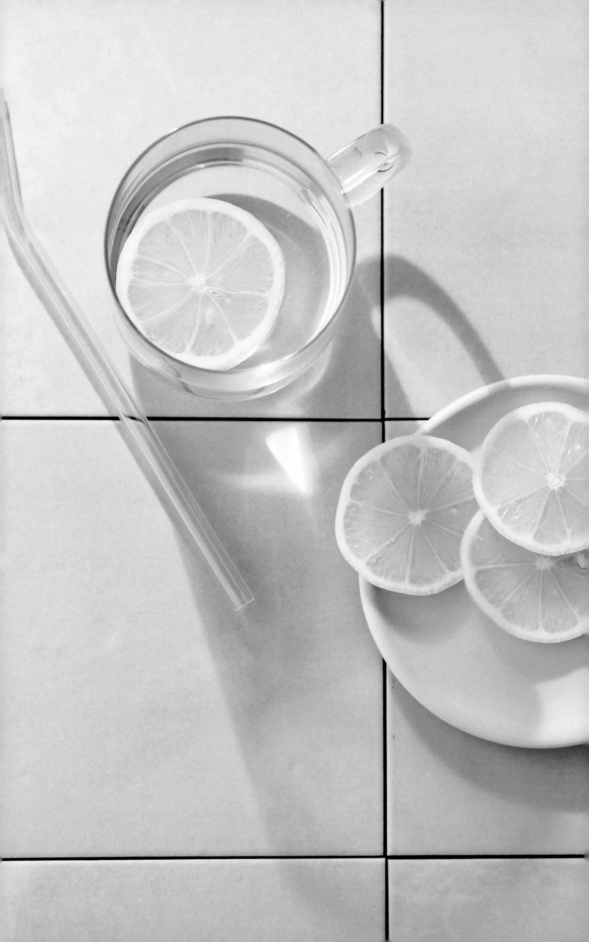

Cauliflower soup

Serves: 4 · Prep: 30 minutes · Cook: 20 minutes

2 tablespoons olive oil

1 large white onion, diced

3 garlic cloves, chopped

1 large head cauliflower, chopped

1 sweet potato, chopped

Sea salt and freshly ground black pepper

2 tablespoons vegetable stock powder

½ cup almond milk

hemp seeds, to serve

Pour the olive oil into a large saucepan over a medium heat. When the oil is hot, stir in the onion and garlic and fry for a couple minutes, until the onion is a pale golden colour and has softened.

Add the cauliflower and sweet potato, then season with sea salt and freshly ground black pepper. Cook, stirring occasionally, for about 5 minutes.

Dissolve the stock powder in 4½ cups of warm water. Pour into the saucepan and bring to the boil. Reduce the heat and simmer for about 10–15 minutes, until the veggies are soft.

Blend the soup using a handheld stick blender (or let it cool slightly, then blend in batches in a blender).

Add the almond milk and blend for just a moment until combined.

If the soup is too thick, add a little more hot water to thin it to the desired consistency.

Ladle into bowls and serve sprinkled with hemp seeds.

Sweet potato salad

Serves: 2 · Prep: 5 minutes · Cook: 30 minutes

1 sweet potato

½ red onion, cut into wedges

olive oil spray

2 handfuls baby spinach leaves

½ punnet cherry tomatoes, halved

2 tablespoons pickled ginger

2 tablespoons sauerkraut

1 tablespoon pumpkin seeds

Coconut aminos, to taste

Optional: 1 avocado, sliced

Preheat the oven to 180°C.

Cut the sweet potato into small cubes. Place on a baking tray with the onion wedges and spray with olive oil. Roast for about 20–25 minutes, until nicely browned, soft and gooey.

Add all the ingredients to a big bowl, gently toss together and serve with avocado, if using.

For a zesty dressing, combine 3 tablespoons lemon juice, 3 tablespoons balsamic vinegar, 1 tablespoon white vinegar, 1 tablespoon olive oil and 2 teaspoons maple syrup.

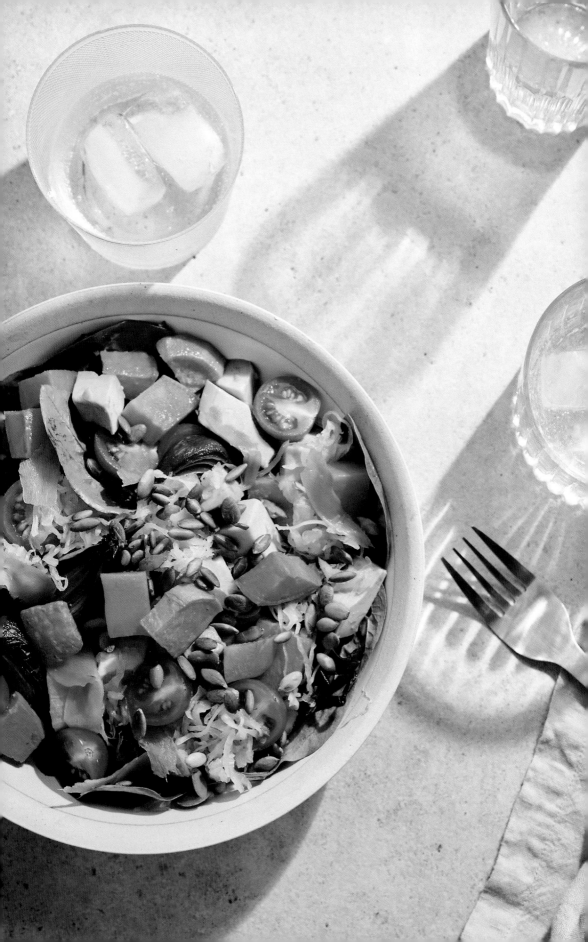

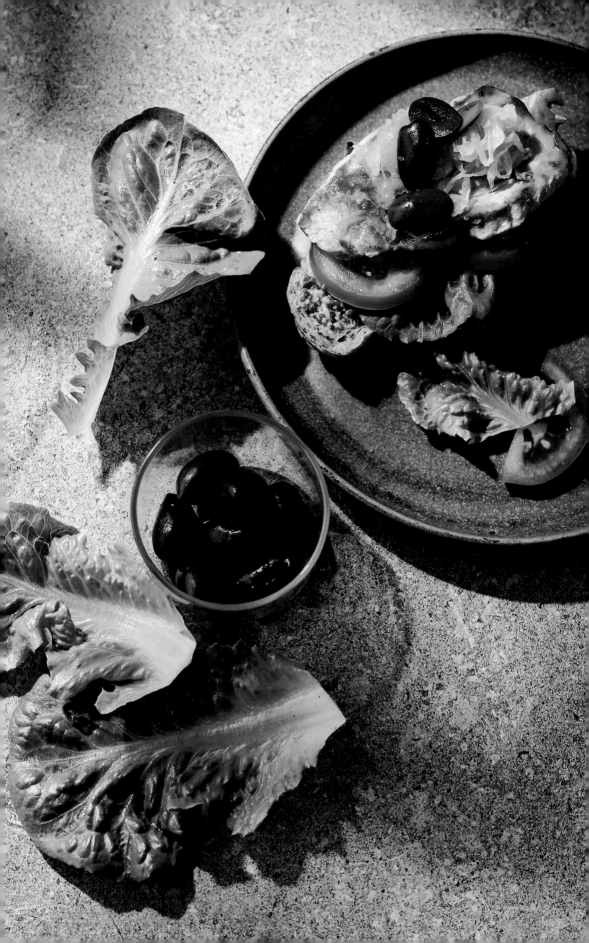

Upside-down pork open sandwiches

Serves: 1 • Prep: 2 minutes • Cook: 5 minutes

100 g pork steak

1 slice multigrain sourdough bread

1 teaspoon butter

1 tablespoon seeded mustard

small handful baby cos lettuce, torn

1 tomato, sliced

2 tablespoons sauerkraut

Optional: 3 black olives, pitted and sliced

Sea salt and freshly ground black pepper

Fry the pork in a frying pan onvera medium–high heat for 1–2 minutes on each side.

Toast the bread and spread with the butter and mustard.

Place on a plate and top with the lettuce, tomato, sauerkraut and olives if you are a fan. Season with sea salt and freshly ground black pepper.

Top with the pork steak and tuck in, using the steak as the sandwich top.

For a bit more sweetness, swap the mustard for an organic barbecue sauce. Personally, olives aren't for me but someone else might like them!

Crunchy chicken salad

Serves: 1 · Prep: 10 minutes

100 g chicken breast, cooked

1 cup green cabbage, finely sliced

3 celery stalks, finely sliced

1 apple, unpeeled and cut into sticks

1 tablespoon pumpkin seeds

2 tablespoons lime juice

1 tablespoon olive oil

Optional: 2 tablespoons pickled ginger

Shred the chicken into pieces and place in a bowl with the cabbage, celery and apple.

Add the pumpkin seeds and mix well.

Drizzle the lime juice and olive oil over the salad, toss together and serve with pickled ginger if using.

You can swap the cabbage for sauerkraut.

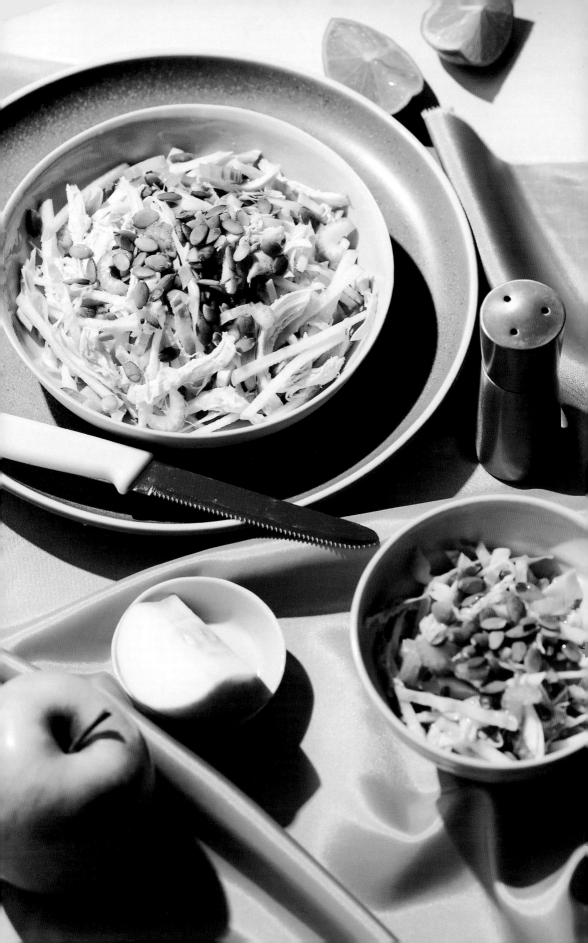

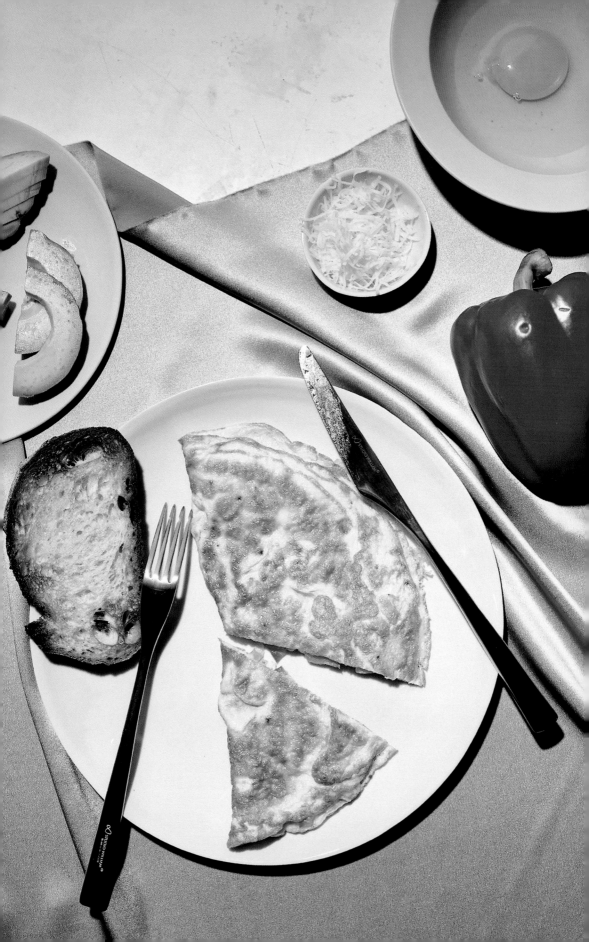

Bone-broth omelette

Serves: 1 • Prep: 2 minutes • Cook: 5 minutes

3 eggs

¼ cup bone broth

¼ red capsicum, finely sliced

¼ cup grated cheese of your choice

1 slice multigrain sourdough, toasted

½ avocado, sliced

Sea salt and freshly ground black pepper

Whisk the eggs with a fork until light and fluffy, then whisk in the bone broth.

Heat a non-stick frying pan over a medium heat and add the egg mixture. After 30 seconds, turn down the heat.

To one half of the omelette, add the capsicum and then the cheese.

Once the omelette is ready, it will start to come away at the sides, after approximately 3–5 minutes. Use a spatula to flip one side onto the other, to create a half-circle.

Finish cooking to the desired consistency.

Serve the omelette straight away on toast, topped with the avocado slices and sprinkled with sea salt and freshly ground black pepper.

I personally don't like avocado, but my husband does, so I keep it on hand for him.

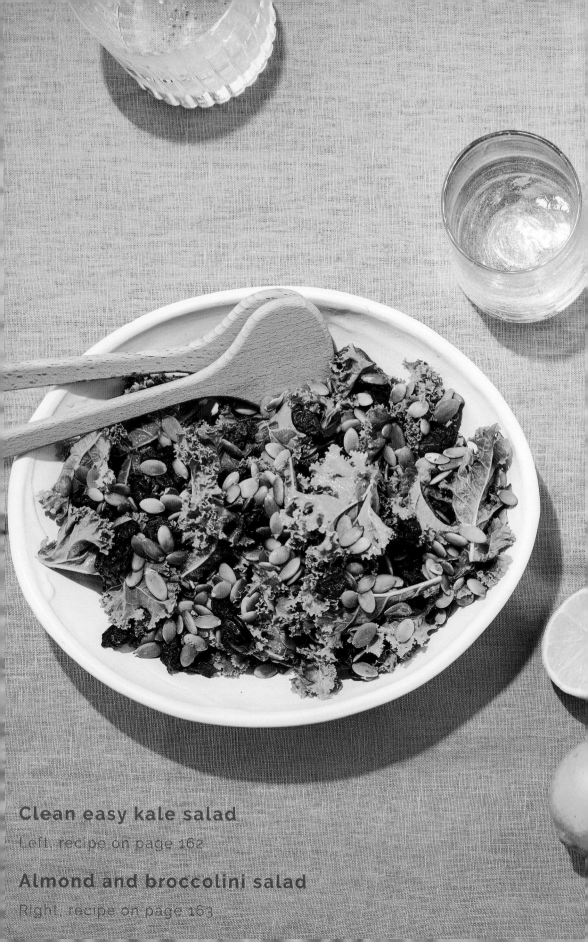

Clean easy kale salad
Left, recipe on page 162

Almond and broccolini salad
Right, recipe on page 163

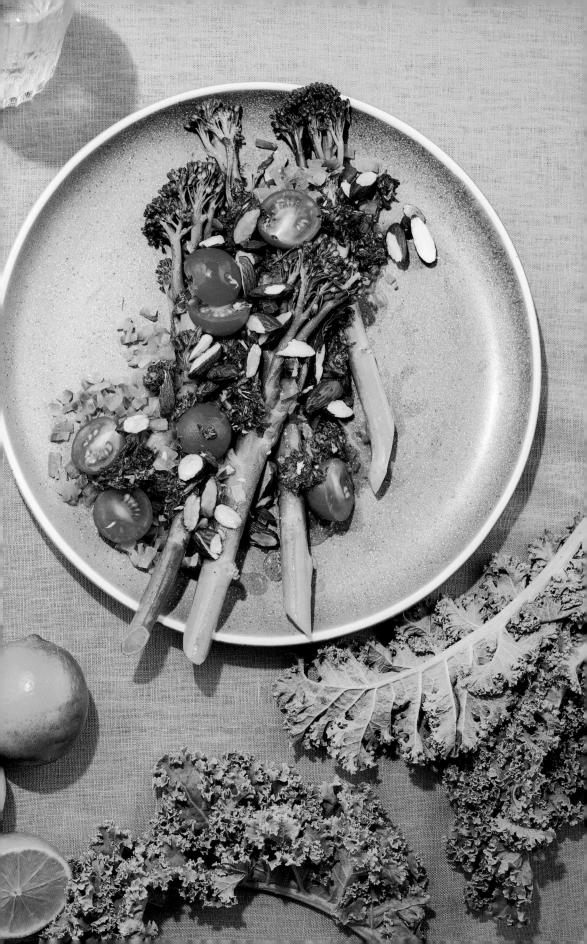

Clean easy kale salad

Serves: 2 • Prep: 5 minutes

1 bunch of kale, leaves roughly torn

1–2 tablespoons olive or coconut oil

¼ cup pumpkin seeds

¼ cup dried cranberries

a squeeze of lemon or lime juice

Optional: 200 g chicken, tofu or sweet potato, cooked

Place the kale leaves in a large bowl and massage in the oil for about 2 minutes, until the kale is soft.

Toss the pumpkin seeds and cranberries through. Drizzle with lemon or lime juice and serve.

Add chicken, tofu or some roasted sweet potato if you'd like to bulk it up.

Massage the oil into the kale a little to soften it - but don't overwork it - this is especially important for large leaves.

Almond and broccolini salad

Serves: 1 • Prep: 5 minutes • Cook: 5 minutes

1 bunch of broccolini, ends trimmed

1 red onion, diced

3 tablespoons olive oil

6 cherry tomatoes, halved

2 tablespoons mixed herbs, such as parsley, coriander, mint and/or chives

2 tablespoons lemon juice

Sea salt and freshly ground black pepper

10 almonds, sliced

Stir-fry the broccolini and onion with 1 tablespoon of olive oil in a hot frying pan or wok over a medium–high heat for 2–4 minutes, until the broccolini is bright green. Make sure the florets still have a crunchy texture.

Once cooked, place the broccolini and onion into a serving bowl, along with the cherry tomatoes.

To make the dressing, add the chopped herbs, 2 tablespoons of olive oil and lemon juice to a separate bowl. Mix well.

Add the dressing to the salad bowl and season with sea salt and freshly ground black pepper. Toss well and sprinkle with almonds to serve.

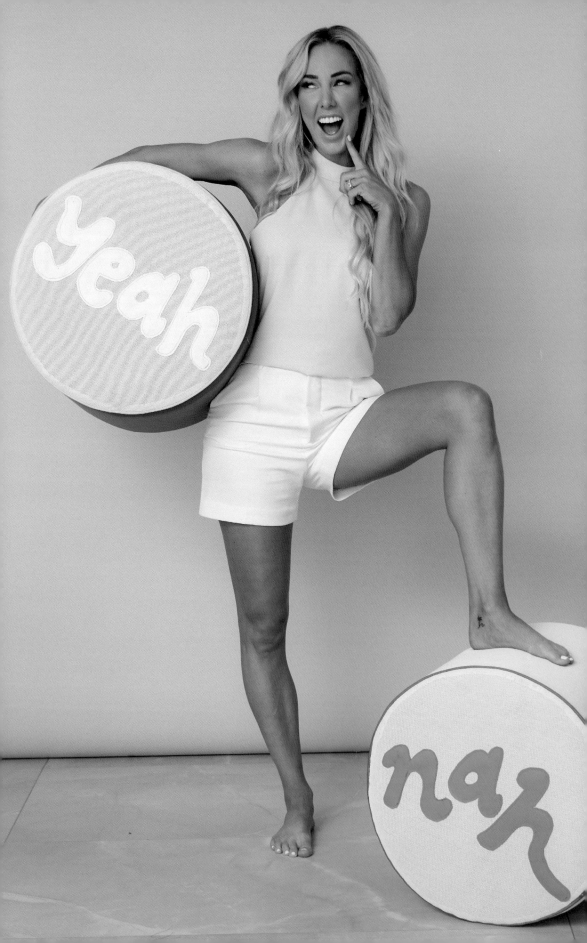

LESSON *Eleven*

♥

There are pros and cons
to everything

LIFE IS A MATTER
OF CHOICES
& EVERY CHOICE
YOU MAKE

makes you

Are you someone who gets really stuck when it comes to making decisions? You're definitely not alone. I know there have been so many times in my own life when I've just felt so unsure about something.

For me, the simple act of writing down the pros and cons of a situation on a piece of paper, or typing them into my notes on my phone, helps me to get clarity and real focus to make the best decision possible.

In life, there will always be tasks that you have to do, or need to do, that you may not enjoy. Even in a relationship, your partner probably has traits that might annoy you or trigger you. However, overall, the positives should outweigh the negatives – and the good times should outweigh the bad times! Otherwise, you probably need to rethink a few things?

As you know, much of what I do in my career happens online. What I love about the online space is that it offers so much opportunity for connection and education, not to mention exciting new possibilities. But as we saw in Lesson Seven, there is also the flip side, the dark side – all the trolling, bullying, negativity, comparing and copying.

Sadly, there have been many times during the past few years when the bad rather than the good has dominated my experience on social media platforms. The barrage of bullying, hateful comments and messages became so overwhelming that they drowned out anything positive. At times, it became so full-on that I felt the need to turn 'off' the comments and put in place a self-imposed 'blackout' week where I could go completely offline. This was an act of self-preservation. It was about taking a break from all the negativity in order to take care of my mental health, to bring my life back into balance, and so the pros had a chance to outweigh the cons.

I haven't felt the need to do this for a long time now, which is a great relief. Yes, for sure, some pretty awful messages and comments still come through – but 90 per cent of them are messages of love and support or are from women wanting advice – which I love, because I love to help!

I'm so happy that these days the good outweighs the small percentage of 'not so nice' in my online interactions.

My husband, Steve, and I have been together for over a decade, and married for more than half of that time. Like all couples, we disagree or argue about things. Even if you are scrolling 'couple goals' and thinking there are 'perfect' couples out there – let me burst that bubble for you here and now.

But, let me also say that for Steve and me, the good always outweighs the hard times.

Yes, we have had times during our years together where the 'hard' has been really hard. There have been times when we were unsure if we would ever resolve a conflict between us or if we even wanted to make any kind of compromise. In those moments, we've really had to ask ourselves if moving forward is the right thing to do, if we are spending more time disconnected from each other and feeling unloved.

I am so very grateful those times didn't last, and that we've always been able to navigate our way through the challenges to reconnect with each other.

Having a relationship coach over the past few years has been incredible! It has helped us to see and understand things from each other's unique perspectives, so that now we are less likely to point the finger and blame. We have more empathy for each other. All of this helps nurture and promote growth in our relationship, even during the challenging times.

There have been many ups and downs during our many years together, and also points when we realised we had both grown so much as individuals. We felt stuck having the same arguments over and over again and not really knowing how to fully resolve them with love and move forward.

We were both being triggered and didn't know how to stop taking the triggers personally. Instead of supporting each other, we'd just end up in an argument, despite knowing in our hearts that it's not who we wanted to be for each other. Old wounds each of us had just hadn't been healed and something needed to be done so that we could remain connected and in love.

We saw a lot of couples fall into becoming just roommates or best friends, and we never wanted that for us, so we knew it was time to get help.

Both of us value our relationship more than anything. I'd been through a lot of therapy and coaching and knew just how much it had helped me to better understand myself, my triggers, my old limiting beliefs, my patterns and generally how I cope and react and respond to certain things.

After watching Tony Robbins help a couple work through their troubles at a course, Steve suggested we find someone to help us do the same. I was so in awe of him for suggesting it, and at the same time excited by the idea of us breaking through some of the barriers that were in our way, so we could ultimately grow together in our relationship.

> *No matter what you're*
> *going through, there is*
> *always someone to help.*

Someone who has experience, knowledge, qualifications, and a genuine concern to contribute, help others and give back to the world to make it a better place.

We never have to do anything alone. There is always someone to help and listen – so why not embrace that help?

When we spend so much time and money on our cars, gym work-outs, healthy food, skin care and so on, why wouldn't we invest as much love and attention on our minds and relationships?

Steve and I spend money on investing in our growth and knowledge, so that we are always learning more and being better people than we were yesterday – both as a couple and as individuals.

LET ME PUT IT LIKE THIS...

Need help with your body? **You hire a personal trainer or nutritionist.**

Need help with a past childhood trauma? **You seek professional advice from a coach or counsellor.**

Need surgery? **Go to a surgeon.**

Have skin issues? **See a beautician or dermatologist.**

Crooked teeth or dental issues? **Visit a dentist.**

Relationship problems or growth? **Hire a relationship coach.**

Pull a muscle? **Physio.**

Back pain? **Chiropractor.**

Falling in love is easy. Staying passionately in love, awake, conscious and deeply connected emotionally, intimately and sexually in your relationship takes mindful actions, energy, time and effort.

Successful marriages and relationships are not accidental – they take work! Yes, you can just be together – but we want to feel love on a deeply connected and passionate level, as well as being each other's best friend.

Ask yourself if there is currently more good than bad/sad in each of these areas? More pros than cons? Where are each of these points leaving you each day? Excited? Sad? Frustrated? Motivated? Giving you purpose?

I really don't believe in perfection; I think the idea of perfection is a false sense of reality and the real world.

I'D LOVE YOU TO DO A BIG, DEEP CHECK-IN WITH THE FOLLOWING THINGS:

♥ Your love relationship (if you aren't currently single)

♥ Friendships

♥ Career/work life

♥ Current health routine

♥ Mindset and the way you show up each day

♥ Self-care/hobbies/fun

But if your energy constantly feels down with a certain person or situation, and you just can't seem to find the joy or look forward to them or the situation, then maybe it's time to make a change?

Change can be uncomfortable at first, but it's where the magic happens.

Without change, we don't grow.

Without growth, we feel dead inside and tend to get stuck – which leads to boredom and lack of purpose and can make it hard to get out of bed some days.

So, that's why these self check-ins are extremely important.

But before you jump in and do anything rash, you might find it helpful to write out a list of the pros and cons. I find it really helpful to see on paper where my thoughts are at – and it honestly just helps to declutter my mind, so I can see clearly what's going on and where I can make some changes to improve my happiness.

Before you make this list, something I love to do first is to go for a walk, take some big breaths, put some nice cruisy music on in the background, make my favourite healthy 'clean treat' and be in a good headspace. This way I don't get stuck on all the negatives and it can be a really enjoyable process writing the list and evaluating where I'm at and where some things can change for me.

Ready to give it a go?

If you look at your list and see there are only one or two pros, but a dozen cons, that's a very clear sign that something or someone is currently not working in your life.

If happiness, mental health, clarity, joy and success are missing, then this person or situation is most likely having a negative impact on more areas of your life than you realise.

So if the cons outweigh the pros – then you know what to do!

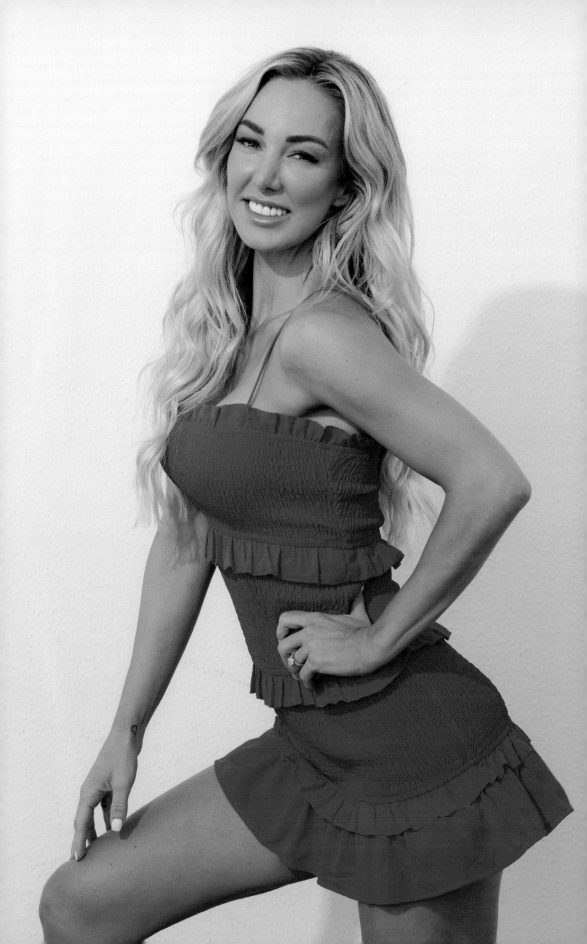

PROS

LOVE RELATIONSHIP

FRIENDSHIPS

CAREER/WORK LIFE

CURRENT HEALTH ROUTINE

MINDSET & THE WAY YOU SHOW UP EACH DAY

SELF-CARE/HOBBIES/FUN

CONS

LOVE RELATIONSHIP

FRIENDSHIPS

CAREER/WORK LIFE

CURRENT HEALTH ROUTINE

MINDSET & THE WAY YOU SHOW UP EACH DAY

SELF-CARE/HOBBIES/FUN

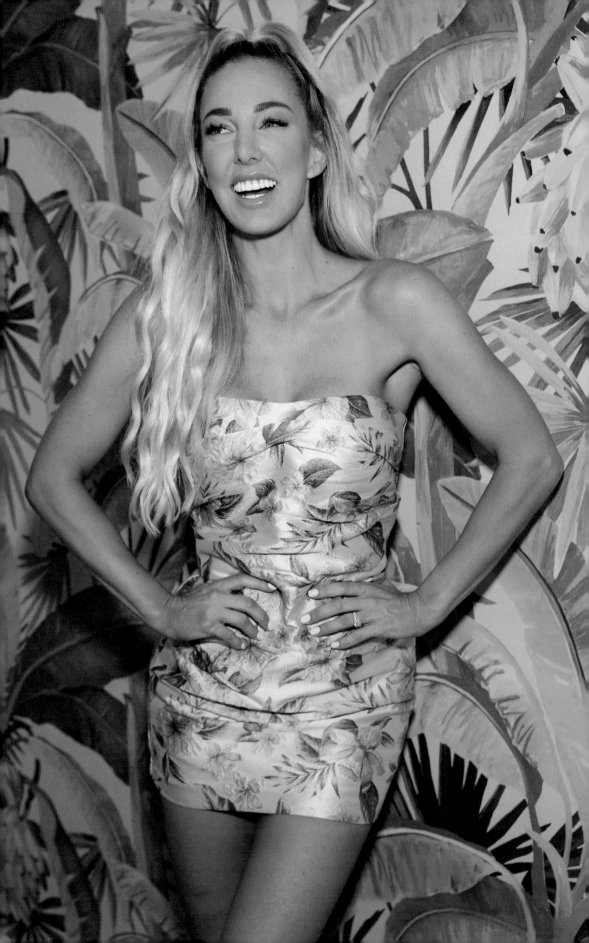

LESSON *twelve*

♥

What you focus on is what you feel

if you

FOCUS ON THE HURT
YOU WILL CONTINUE
TO SUFFER

if you

FOCUS ON THE
LESSON YOU WILL
CONTINUE TO GROW

Ever had a day where you feel like crap? Is it hard to stop thinking about how crap you feel? And how crap life feels? And how there are so many crappy things in your life right now? And then you just feel like an even bigger pile of crap? Literally? LOL.

Or have you ever felt just so happy?

Then sat and thought about how friggin' happy you feel?

How happy you are about all the great people around you?

And how there are so many awesome things happening in your life?

You can't stop smiling about it all and that makes you feel even more happy?

This goes to show that whatever feelings you focus on will expand.

If you keep focusing on the good, the bad, the upset, the gratitude, the happiness – whatever it is that you are feeling – it will just get bigger and bigger. Your heart and your mind will lock onto that feeling and will elevate and expand it.

So if we're having positive feelings, they can work in our favour – and when we're feeling negative, sad emotions, they aren't going to be serving us well at all.

Now, I'm definitely not saying you should ignore any feelings of sadness or frustration or anger that arise, because I strongly believe it's very important to feel them all. But you really do have to ask yourself how LONG you want to be feeling them and question whether they are actually SERVING you – or is there a way to switch the feelings around so you can move through them and they don't become bigger or worse than they need to be?

When I was 19 and going through depression, all I would think about and focus on all of the time was how depressed and sad I was feeling.

I would tell myself over and over again that I'd never be happy, that I'd never make anything of myself and that no one would ever love me. That's ALL I was putting out into the Universe. I almost made it my mantra!

So guess what I was attracting into my life?

Love? No.

Happiness? No.

Opportunities? Nope.

All I was doing was calling in even more negativity and more sadness to fuel my depression. I didn't even try to change or shift the state I was in – I just moped around and spiralled deeper and deeper downwards. The sadness eventually felt so comfortable that it became my emotional home. In some messed-up way, it also brought me a lot of love, attention and connection with those around me – all the things I felt starved of while growing up. But this was not doing me any favours and was definitely not healthy on any level. Nor did it really give me the relationships and connections I knew I wanted, because every conversation was about how sad I was.

Thinking back to this time, it seems that when I felt most depressed, I was also the most selfish I had ever been. There was no room in my own head or heart to think about anyone else. All I could think about was how depressed I was. Yes, there were valid reasons for why I was struggling, but I also never focused on anything positive – and there actually WERE positives in my life during that period.

Nor did I consider that there were people worse off than me. Being here with two feet and a heartbeat means I'm bloody lucky. But let's continue on with going down that depressive spiral.

Hitting rock bottom can actually be a good thing, in a surreal way, because once you're down as far as you can go – the only way is up! Looking back, it wasn't one moment or one book or one person that snapped me out of my bleakness – it happened over time. I began looking after myself, including my physical health and my mental health, more and more, which impacted on my view of the world and my happiness.

After I started to feel better, happier, more motivated, I became addicted to feeling good. By 'addicted', I mean that in the most healthy and positive way. It made me want to chase those 'feel-good' feelings.

I was no longer interested in having people connect with me only because I was sad and they pitied me or because they wanted to save me and make my pain disappear. I wanted to connect with them on my own terms – for who I was NOW and not the person I had been.

It also made me want to focus on HOW I could bring more happiness, more positivity and more connection to others.

It worked in shifting my awareness so that I thought more about others, rather than just focusing on me and what I was going through.

I decided I wanted to be someone people loved to be around. I wanted to be that person who brings a sense of happiness and lightness when they walk into a room. I wanted to make everybody feel like a somebody!

It made me realise how important it was to make a positive impact on people's lives – every single day of my life. I also understood that this required me to do the work on myself. It was unrealistic that anyone else would be inspired to change their own lives and work on themselves if I hadn't done the work on myself first.

EVERY single day we get to choose what we focus on. Since we have thousands of thoughts and feelings every single day, let's make a real effort to choose and focus on the ones that bring us real joy and happiness.

Let's also promise to spread that joy and happiness around to those around us. It's infectious – in a good way!

Even if you find you can't do that every day, then remember the first step to changing is being aware. So it's about catching yourself when you find yourself slipping back into any negative thought patterns or starting to feel like the victim. PAUSE! Catch it, breathe into it, lean into it and then you're already back on a positive track, so that the next move you make and the next action you take are ones that make you FEEL GOOD – or at least better! – and serve you and others.

It's the reason Lesson One of this book is so important to me – because when we focus on gratitude, it brings happiness and the feeling that the glass is always half full, rather than half empty.

And it can't hurt to give you just another reminder that you can't be grateful and angry at the same time.

MY THREE TIPS ON SHIFTING MINDSET

1 **MOVE your body.** This is always my number-one thing to do to change my state, change my mood, get those endorphins going and get my head nice and clear so I can have the energy and positive mind frame to get done what I need to do. Remember, I'm not talking about smashing yourself in the gym every day – I mean a nice walk along the beach, an at-home workout, maybe some stair sprints or a yoga session ... whatever movement feels good for YOU!

2 **Eat GOOD nutritious FOOD.** I'm a massive foodie and I don't know too many people who don't have a love of food. Grocery shopping for food, being in the kitchen preparing food, trying the food, serving the food to my loved ones – the entire process just makes me feel good inside! Especially knowing it's clean, nutritious, healthy food. Knowing I'm doing something good for my loved ones' health makes me so SO happy and is such a perfect way to shift my mood and change my state. Try it!

3 **Remember SELF-CARE.** All of us are guilty of not always giving ourselves the self-care and love we need and deserve. Why is it that we feel so guilty about taking care of ourselves? I have well and truly let go of feeling any guilt when it comes to looking after myself. WHAT, WHY, HOW, you are asking? It's actually pretty simple. By looking after myself, I can then look after others. Being both a mum and wife, I always want to take care of my family – but I can't do that without taking care of myself. So, they are in fact my motivation and reason to let go of the guilt. Plus, own it! Girl, you work hard, give SO much and you bloody deserve a hot bath with a gorgeous-smelling bath bomb while you've got that hair and face mask soaking in and a cup of tea by your side!

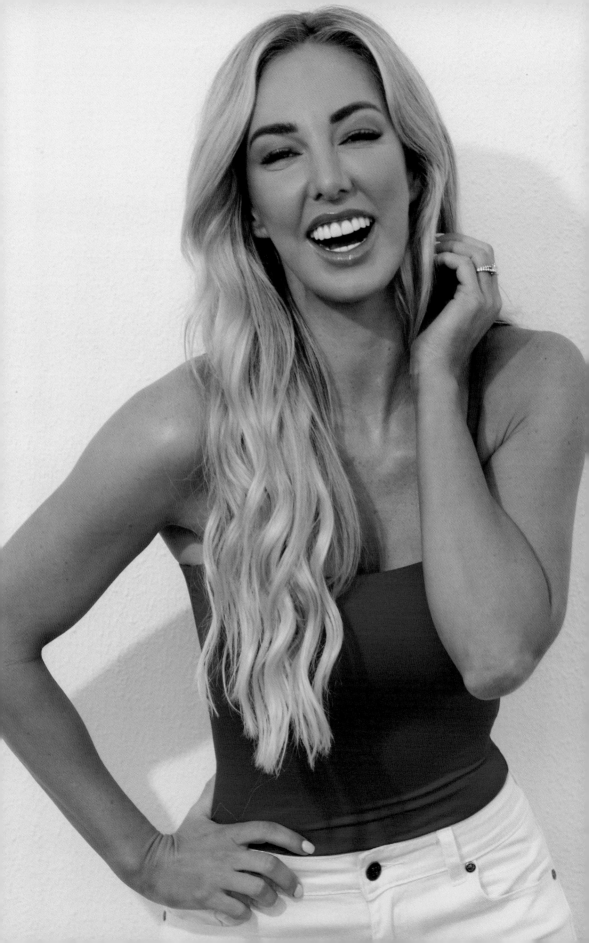

LESSON *Thirteen*

♥

Everything passes.
Nothing lasts forever

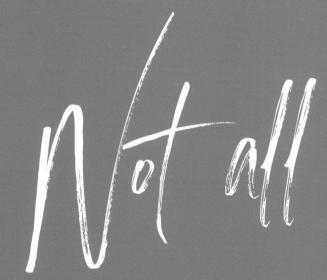

Not all

STORMS COME TO
DISRUPT YOUR LIFE

Sometimes when we go through something really hard and challenging, we can get so stuck inside our heads and wonder, 'When will this ever end?' or 'Is this how it's going to be forever?'

But we have to remember that nothing really lasts forever, and everything is just a passing phase in our lives. Sometimes these times may go on longer than we'd like or want – but knowing that they're only temporary can help to reduce the stress while we're going through them.

When I look back to the early days when my beautiful son Taj was just a newborn, it honestly felt like I was never going to get a full night's sleep, ever again. I'd get so anxious every evening, knowing I'd be woken up in just a few hours to feed him again and to calm his crying. I hate admitting this, because I do know just how damn lucky I am to have a child. Trust me, I don't take it for granted, ever. But I want to be honest with you and tell you that I really struggled with the newborn stage.

I was seriously scared that I'd never be able to sleep through the night again, never be able to eat by myself, that my back would never get a break from carrying this chubby, clingy child of mine. It was also physically tough. I was in pain from constantly carrying him, my boobs were always sore and my whole body had a lot of healing to do after the birth, which I found scary and overwhelming.

At the same time, yes, I did embrace every single cuddle, and felt so lucky that I was the one responsible for giving him comfort and relieving his pain. But I'm not going to lie and tell you it was easy. It was not!

If only someone had reassured me then that this wouldn't last forever and that the newborn stage is just a phase, just like the toddler phase and just like each and every stage and age kids transition through.

Yes, in hindsight that was obvious and logical, but through the lens of a sleep-deprived, emotional, hormone-surged first-time new mum – it just was not! My emotions were in the driver's seat and I was trying hard to just survive, so I couldn't really think clearly enough to understand that this, too, would pass.

A different moment in my life where I struggled to focus beyond the 'now' was when I was experiencing the surge of online hate. You would have read earlier in this book just how much it really affected me – much more than I can even put into words. But yet again, it was just a phase in my life – and although I thought it would never end, I really, really wish back then that I could have realised that the intensity of it was not going to last forever.

When it comes to my work, I sometimes feel overwhelmed because I'm being pulled by too many people or because we have too many projects on the go simultaneously. But once again, it's only a phase, and in fact when things start to get slower and quieter, I actually start to get excited about getting busy again!

Knowing that nothing lasts forever, we need to start being more flexible and learn how to flow with the ups and downs in life.

Once we master that, then our lives will generally become a lot less stressful – and way more enjoyable. Being more in tune with our bodies and our cycles is also key, as these can really impact our emotions, energy and our clarity. Tapping into those cycles stops us from getting so caught up in life's challenging moments.

So, the next time you find yourself having those conversations in your head about 'When is this all going to end?', I'd like you to stop and take ten big breaths.

Then remind yourself that this crazy, busy or challenging chapter in your life is a temporary phase – it won't always be like this.

Do your very best to get through it,
find gratitude in the busyness and reach out
for help as much as you need!

It's not possible to wave a magic wand and make it all disappear, but you definitely can 'do what you can do' and be okay about letting go of what can wait until tomorrow – or even next week.

Remember – it's only a phase! You can only do what you can. Meanwhile, you literally just need to DO YOU.

Better days are on the way.

KEEP CALM
BECAUSE

nothing

LASTS
FOREVER

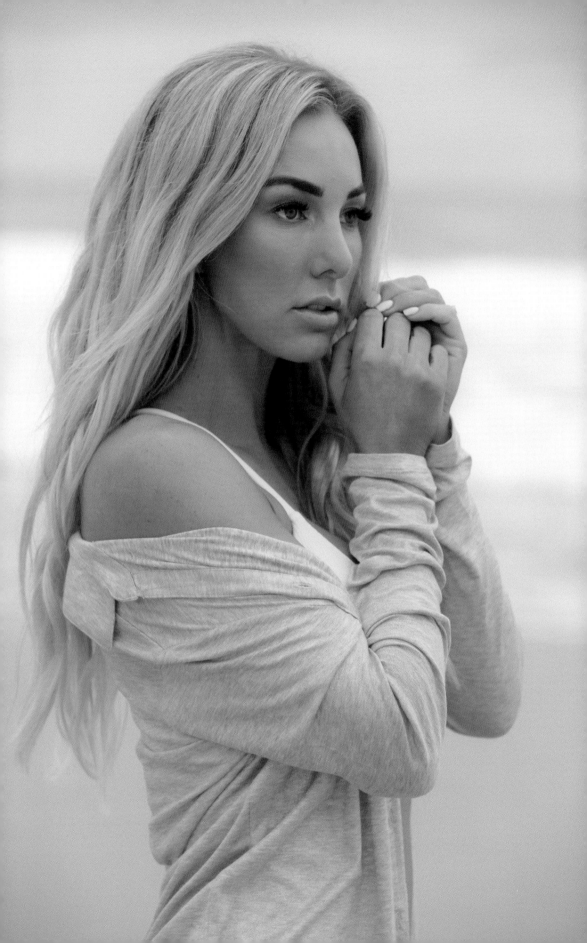

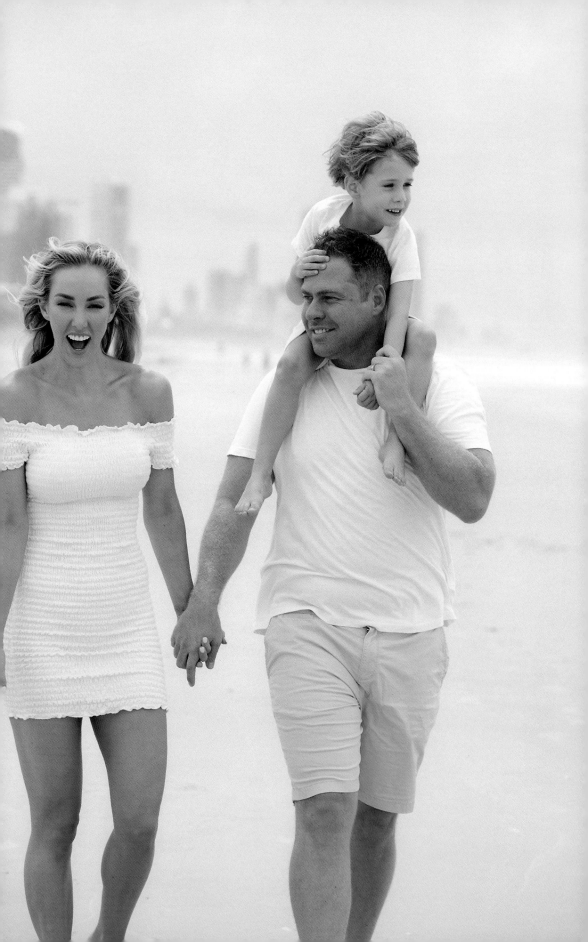

LESSON *Fourteen*

♥

Balance. Always find
time for the things that
make you happy

THE KEY
IS NOT TO
PRIORITISE
WHAT'S
ON YOUR
SCHEDULE
BUT TO

schedule
your priorities

This is a topic I am SO excited to chat to you about, because it's something I talk about ALL the time. Some people don't believe the idea of balance is even a real thing. Now, I'm not saying it's always easy to find balance in our lives these days, but I do think it's possible.

There are so many things that you love doing, right?

So many things you need to do?

So many people to see who you enjoy being around, who light you up?

So many tasks to do that are important for your health, your family and your life?

I get it. I get that for many of us life is tough, and a lot of people say, 'Well, *you just can't have it all.*'

Well, I'm calling that out for what it is – BULLSHIT!
WHY CAN'T WE HAVE IT ALL?

Who said we can't? Who made that rule? Why are we all going along with it? Why are we settling for second best? Is it simply because society or someone is telling us we can't have it all?

No thanks! I have my own vision for the kind of life I want to live. I plan on being extremely happy by doing things that are fun and help me feel alive, feel connected and feel young.

The way I see it is that if there are certain things, tasks, activities, people, foods that make me happy and that I enjoy – I'd like to figure out how can I have them all in my life!

First up, I want you to write down what it is that makes you happy and what you'd love to enjoy each week. Don't worry about how you're going to do that just yet. Don't think about the 'how' right now. Just list what those things are for you on page 199.

Let me share mine with you so you can understand how I make it happen for me.

FAMILY

Quality time with my family every week is so important to me. I'm always conscious that parents and older family members aren't going to be around forever, so spending quality time with them, especially my mum, is so very important. If you have kids and/or a partner, maintaining that connection with extended family is especially important. Life just isn't the same if you aren't able to share it with those you care about and who care about you.

FRIENDS

I always need and love my girlfriends. Yes, I find it gets harder to find time together as we get older, for sure, but they are still a priority for me. That connection we feel and get from our girlfriends is really special. All that sharing and opening up to each other, being there for each other's ups and downs is intense and wonderful at the same time.

FOOD

Eating out and socialising is definitely my 'thing'. Plus I just love discovering and experiencing new foods! I love the variety, the memories it creates … and did I say that I really enjoy food!?

FITNESS

Training time is also my ME time. For me, training is my biggest stress relief and outlet. It is so helpful to my mental health – more than I can even explain. Feeling strong in the gym helps me feel strong mentally and emotionally. I notice such a big difference in my week if I don't make time for health and fitness and moving my body.

ME TIME

I need pockets of time for me to ground, to chill, to recharge. I always want to be the best version of me, so I can give everyone and everything the best of me – not the rest of me. This also happens to be my favourite quote for self-care!

FUN TIME

I love planning adventures, including variety in what I do and finding something different and new that excites me. Or even just remembering to enjoy and do the things that make me smile and laugh. What's life if we aren't having fun, right?

WORK

I really do love what I do! Let's face it, we all need to work, so work is a must for us to fit into our lives and always needs to be a priority.

So now that we have our list, it's really as simple as just scheduling it all in. So let's do it!

I do believe that creating structure around most of the things we do gives us a far better chance of actually making them happen. Too often, things get busy, work takes over and other parts of your life that are important to you end up taking a back seat. But if you neglect those other parts of your life, I can guarantee that you won't feel as happy or as whole as you could feel – and should feel!

I love routine. Actually, I absolutely thrive on routine. Now, that doesn't mean I'm not flexible. I can 100 per cent be flexible – but I also want everyone reading this book who thinks that I always perfectly balance my life to know that this is not always the reality.

Even the writing deadline for this book meant that completing this project became my main focus for a few weeks, which unbalanced some other parts of my life, such as seeing my friends, for instance. But I do know how to get back into balance and I always feel best when I go back to the routine that works for me, because in some sense the structure of that makes me happy.

If you are planning your wedding, for example, health and fitness may become a huge priority, so that you can look and feel your best on your big day. If that's the case, then socialising may no longer be such a big priority or you simply get creative when it comes to connecting and catching up with friends. That might mean you invite them over and cook dinner for them instead of eating out.

Yes, it's all about planning and having structure – but it's also about embracing the unpredictability of life, so we can adapt our mindset when needed.

AND don't forget about being really kind to ourselves along the way and through the different seasons of our lives. We need to accept change and learn to be okay with it when life doesn't always go to our plan.

Ironically, while I was writing this lesson, I didn't really feel very balanced. There was a huge work meeting in Brisbane that I absolutely had to show up for and which couldn't be rescheduled. That meant I would miss out on my weekly all-day 'Mummy Day'. This is a day where I try to put all my work commitments aside and my son Taj doesn't go to day care, so that we get to spend the entire day together.

It's such a very special time for both of us, so it's very rare that I allow anything to impact on our day together. But sometimes you just have no choice. I made sure to free up the following Tuesday for Taj, and I let my team know that I would be unavailable.

Things may not always go to plan, but if we schedule in what is important to us and what makes us happy, then most of the time we won't be missing out or feeling deprived of things and people. Our cup will be full and we'll be feeling pretty damn happy with life, because we're getting to enjoy all the things we love.

A lot of the time, the pressure we feel to be perfect and have everything perfect or do things in a certain perfect way comes mostly from the pressure we put on ourselves. Try sitting with that feeling and ask yourself why you are feeling like that? I find much of the time I'm putting that pressure on myself. Is that true for you, too?

There are no rules on how things have to be in your life. You can go and ask people you trust or people you love learning from or listen to whatever podcast inspires you. But it's up to you to find out what works for you.

Please just remember to be KIND to yourself while you're trying to figure it all out...

WHAT MAKES YOU HAPPY?

What things would you like to enjoy every week? Write down everything you can think of.

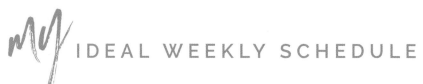 IDEAL WEEKLY SCHEDULE

This is a very general outline of my week. Please know that some weeks are crazy and it's all Baseline-focused, while other weeks I get more time with Taj. Sometimes I'll record back-to-back podcasts as it's the only timeslot I can get with the guest. So, yes, I'm structured – but in a flexible way.

MONDAY

Stretch and walk, drop Taj at day care then head to the office to meet my team for a debrief. As well as being a big admin day, I also work across all my different projects like my Baseline label and our Transform app, I film content, have Hideaway or Clean Treats meetings and review other brand enquiries.
It's when I plan questions for my Raw and Real podcast series and outline my social media content for the week. Visiting the Baseline warehouse in Brisbane for design meetings and fittings is also usually on the agenda.

TUESDAY

My day with my son Taj. A slow start with cuddles in bed followed by a long walk, stopping at different parks, a healthy breakfast together and then off to his gymnastics class. After a cute lunch together when we get home, he has his day sleep from 12–2pm. During this time I usually record a podcast, after which I'll go straight back to spending quality time with my little man.

WEDNESDAY

Stretch, walk, and train then home to make a protein smoothie and take Taj to day care. Usually I'll head to the office for a few hours work with my personal assistant for more meetings and to plan content. Once we wrap I like to take her out for a Cocowhip or açaí bowl and some quality time together. Although it may not happen every week, I aim to book in an appointment with my chiropractor, acupuncturist or maybe get a skin treatment. It's just a little something for my wellbeing that I look forward to. Driving to Brisbane for Baseline meetings is also a possibility, but I try to have these over Skype so I can have more home time with Taj and Steve. My team are incredible and do their jobs so well there's no need for micro-managing.

THURSDAY

Stretch and 45-minute walk, followed by a few hours in the office. I usually film a video for my YouTube channel. I love thinking about and planning these as I want my videos to feature content that really helps women in some way. I set aside Thursday nights for a weekly date night with my besties so we can catch up and stay connected. We get dinner, usually followed by ice-cream. It's our special night and I really look forward to getting together with them.

FRIDAY

Walk and train, plus my stretch routine. Today is usually a big day of photo shoots, filming for Baseline or friends' brands if they want help. I LOVE pulling together inspiring content for my social media. This is a day for me to reflect back on the week and review and revise my schedule for the following week. Taj and I love to pop in on my mum in the afternoon to spend time with her. It's such a nice way to end the work week.

SATURDAY

We aim not to have too many plans for the weekend. We start the day with some kind of movement, followed by breakfast, and then a swim at the beach. While Taj has his midday sleep, Steve and I catch up on emails, messages and calls, then watch a movie and chill. Tonight's our weekly date night. We love staying connected and being able to have a conversation without Taj interrupting every three seconds! Either my mum, Steve's mum or a babysitter looks after Taj so we can make sure we get this time together every week.
It's so important to both of us.

SUNDAY

Sundays are chill! I go to the beach, do my grocery shopping and food prep for the week. I like to go over my upcoming schedule and plan meetings, shoots and social media content, and create a checklist to go over with my team on Monday so I can plan for a productive week ahead!

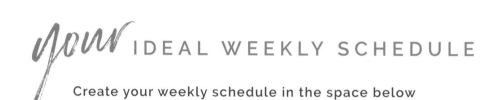

your IDEAL WEEKLY SCHEDULE

Create your weekly schedule in the space below

MONDAY

TUESDAY

WEDNESDAY

THURSDAY

FRIDAY

SATURDAY

SUNDAY

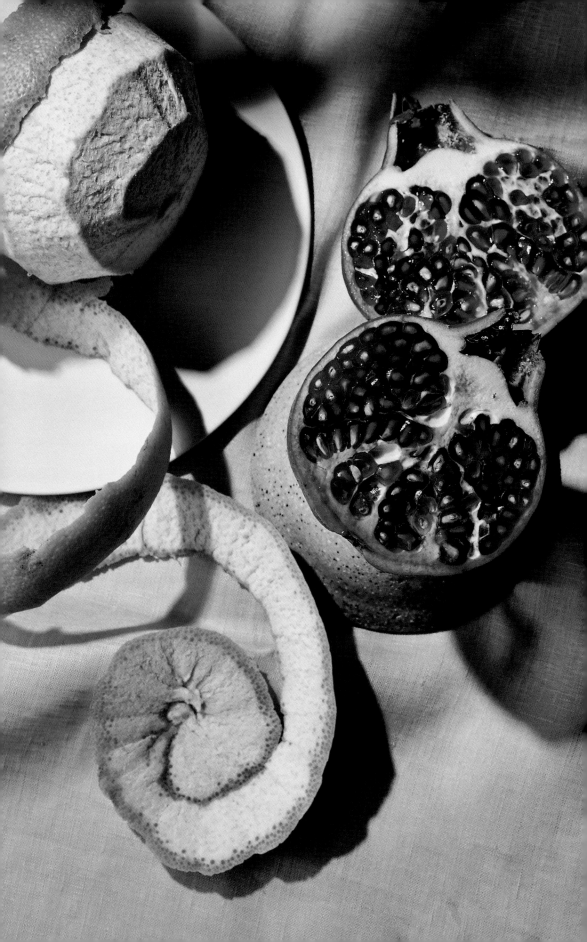

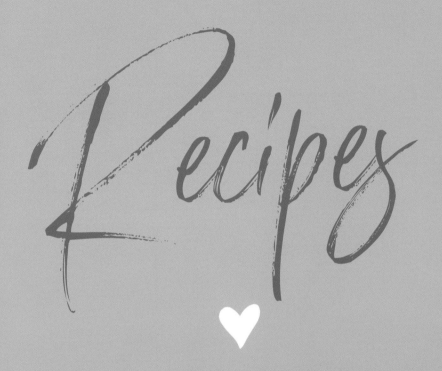

Recipes

♥

DINNERS & DESSERTS

At the end of a busy day, I want
fuss-free, healthy meals that I
can whip up in a flash and that
everyone will enjoy

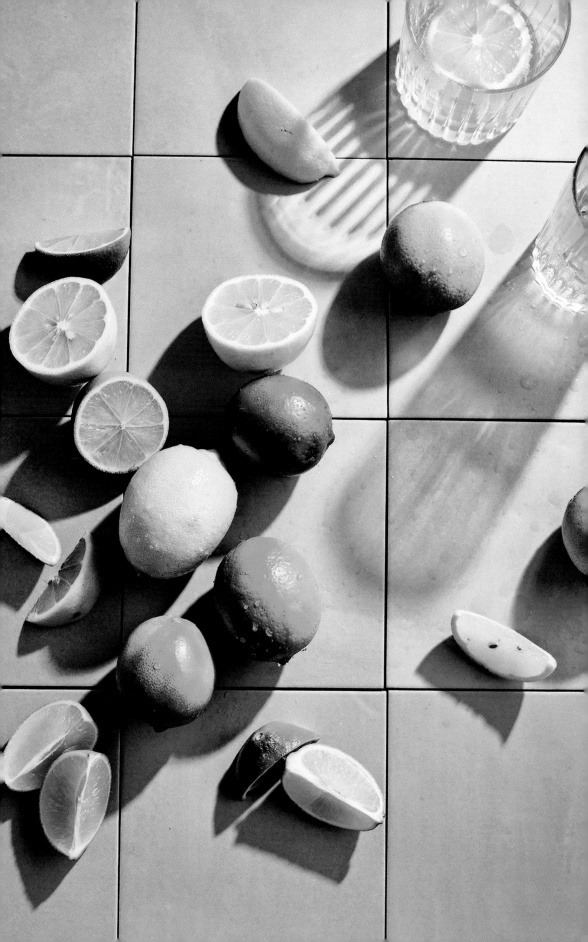

Savoury mince bliss

Serves: 1 · Prep: 10 minutes · Cook: 20 minutes

1 teaspoon extra virgin olive oil

¼ red onion, diced

200 g lean minced beef (5 per cent fat)

1 teaspoon cumin seeds

Sea salt and freshly ground black pepper

1½ tablespoons tomato paste

½ carrot, sliced

1 garlic clove, crushed

1 red chilli, finely sliced

Baby spinach leaves, to serve

Heat a small non-stick frying pan over a medium–high heat. Add the olive oil and onion and cook over a low heat for about 5 minutes or until translucent.

Add the beef mince and cumin seeds, and season with sea salt and freshly ground black pepper. Continue cooking for 10 minutes, breaking up the mince as you go.

Stir in the tomato paste, carrot, garlic and chilli until combined. Add 1 tablespoon of water and cook for a further 5 minutes.

Serve on a bed of baby spinach.

Loaded cauli fried rice

Serves: 1 · Prep: 2 minutes · Cook: 8 minutes

1 cup cauliflower florets

2 teaspoons virgin cold-pressed coconut oil

1 egg, beaten

150 g lean middle bacon rashers, diced

¼ red onion, diced

1 garlic clove, crushed

4 brussels sprouts, halved

1 tablespoon tamari

chopped parsley, to serve

In a food processor or using a knife, chop the cauliflower until a texture like rice is achieved. Set aside.

Heat the coconut oil in a frying pan over a medium heat. Add the egg to the pan and cook for 2 minutes, or until set. Remove from the pan, slice into strips and set aside.

In the same pan, add the bacon and cook for 2 minutes. Add the onion and garlic. Cook for a further 2 minutes, until translucent. Add the brussels sprouts and cook for a further 2 minutes, stirring occasionally. These can also be cooked and served separately for picky eaters!

Add the cauliflower rice and tamari and toss until all the ingredients are evenly coated with tamari.

Serve immediately, sprinkled with parsley.

For a spicy version, add fresh chilli or dried chilli flakes.

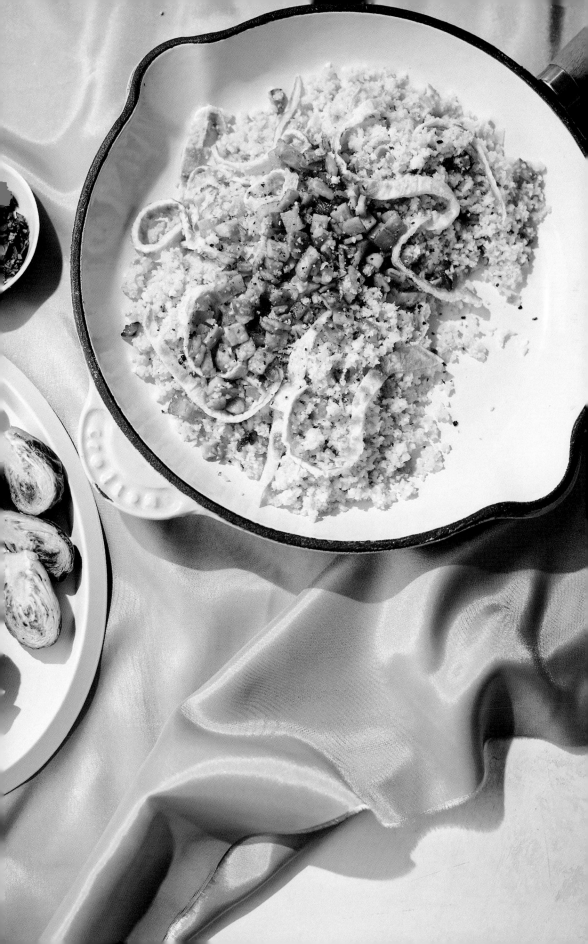

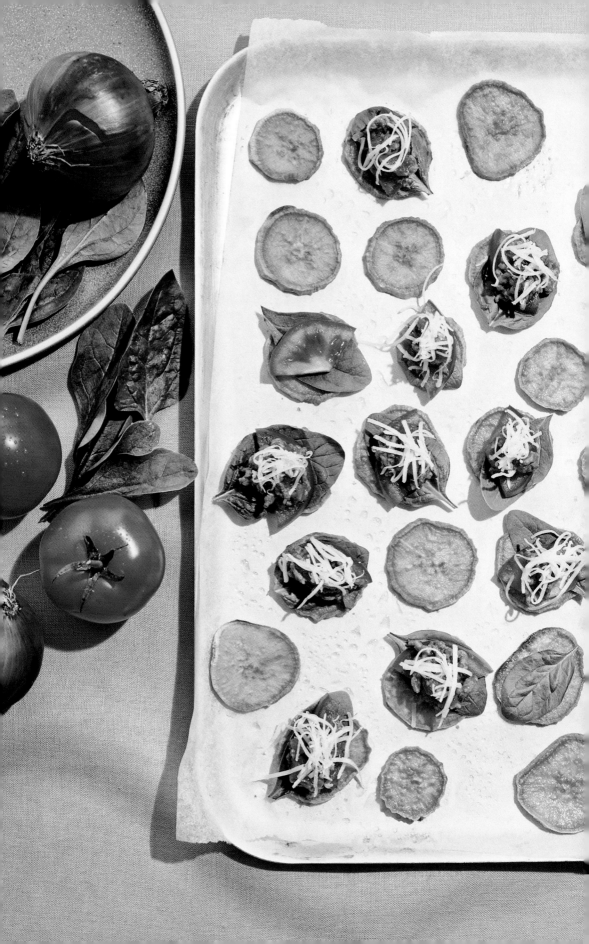

Sweet potato nachos

Serves: 2-3 · Prep: 20 minutes · Cook: 30 minutes

1 sweet potato, cut into 5 mm thick slices

olive oil spray

1 tablespoon olive oil

1 onion, diced

500 g lean minced beef (5 per cent fat)

500 g tinned tomatoes

1 cup baby spinach leaves

1 tomato, finely sliced

¼ cup grated cheese of your choice

Sea salt and freshly ground black pepper

Preheat the oven to 180°C. Line a baking tray with baking paper.

Place the sweet potato slices on the baking tray, spray with oil and bake for 20 minutes, turning them over after 10 minutes.

Meanwhile, place the olive oil and the onion in a frying pan and cook over a medium–low heat for about 2 minutes, until translucent. Add the beef mince and cook for about 5 minutes, until browned, breaking up the lumps as you go. Stir in the tinned tomatoes and simmer for a further 5 minutes.

Remove the baking tray from the oven. Place a baby spinach leaf on each sweet potato slice, then top with a tomato slice. Spoon a layer of the sauce on top, sprinkle with cheese and season with sea salt and freshly ground black pepper.

To increase your veggie intake, you can add corn kernels and/or grated beetroot to your nachos.

Zucchini turkey pesto

Serves: 1 · Prep: 5 minutes · Cook: 5 minutes

1 zucchini

olive oil spray

½ red onion, chopped

3 garlic cloves, chopped

100 g minced turkey

3–4 tablespoons basil pesto

¼ cup grated or sliced parmesan

Use a julienne slicer or spiraliser to make noodles from the zucchini.

Place a saucepan over a medium heat and spray with olive oil. Add the onion and garlic and cook for about 2–3 minutes, until golden brown.

Add the turkey mince and cook for about 5 minutes, stirring occasionally, until the turkey is cooked.

Toss in the zucchini noodles and pesto and mix them through.

Serve immediately, topped with the parmesan.

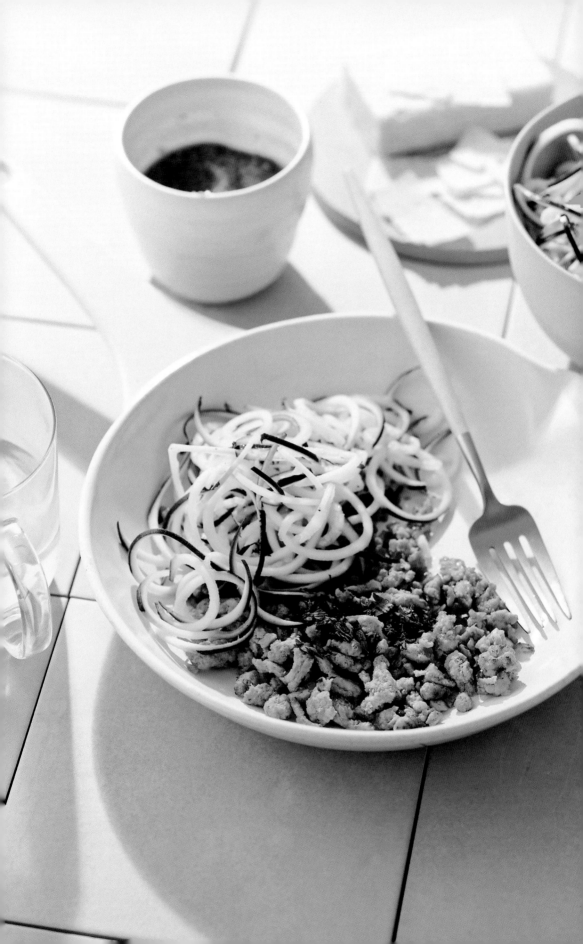

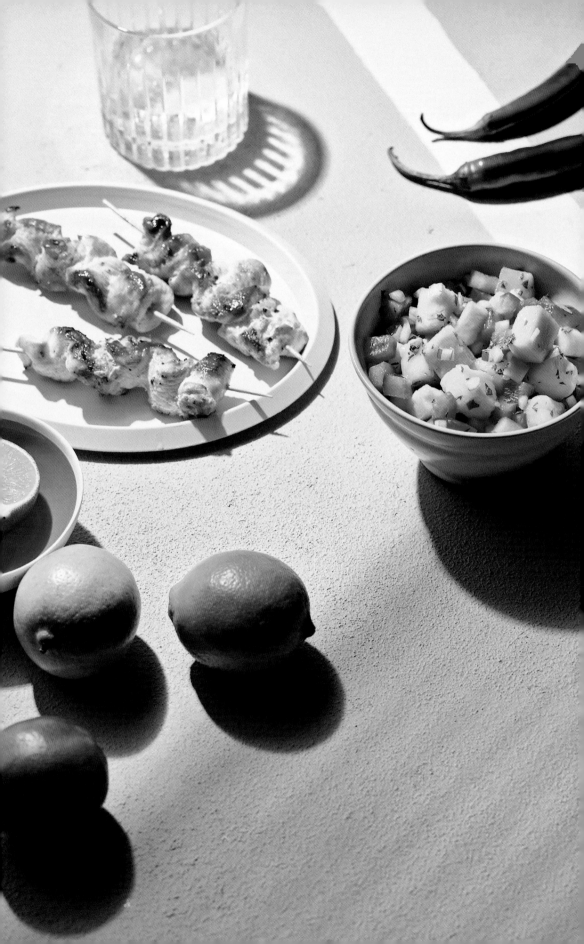

Mum's mango salsa

Serves: 2 · Prep: 5 minutes

Flesh of 1–2 large ripe mangoes, diced

½ red capsicum, finely diced

⅓ red onion, finely chopped

½ teaspoon finely chopped red or green chilli (or to taste)

1 small handful of chopped coriander

Sea salt and freshly ground black pepper

Juice of 1 lime

1 teaspoon fish sauce

Optional:

Chopped parsley, basil or mint

⅓ cup corn kernels

⅓ cup diced cucumber

Put the mango, capsicum, onion, chilli and coriander into a large bowl, along with any optional extras. Season with sea salt and freshly ground black pepper.

Mix together the lime juice and fish sauce, then drizzle over the salsa.

Gently toss together and serve immediately, sprinkled with parsley, if using. This salsa is great with BBQ chicken skewers!

Sweet potato stir-fry

Serves: 2 • Prep: 5 minutes • Cook: 10 minutes

2 tablespoons coconut oil

2 large sweet potatoes, cut into rounds

1 red onion, cut into wedges

Sea salt and freshly ground black pepper

2 cups baby spinach leaves

2 teaspoons coconut aminos, plus extra to serve

1 cup coriander leaves

toasted sesame seeds, to serve

toasted pumpkin seeds, to serve

Heat the coconut oil in a large saucepan or wok. Add the sweet potato and onion and stir until coated with oil. Season with sea salt and freshly ground black pepper, then cover with a lid and cook over a medium heat for about 5–7 minutes, stirring occasionally; add more coconut oil if it starts to stick.

When the sweet potato is almost soft, stir in the spinach and coconut aminos. Put the lid back on for a few minutes, until the spinach has wilted.

Remove from the heat and stir the coriander through.

Serve sprinkled with toasted sesame and pumpkin seeds, and a dash more of coconut aminos if needed.

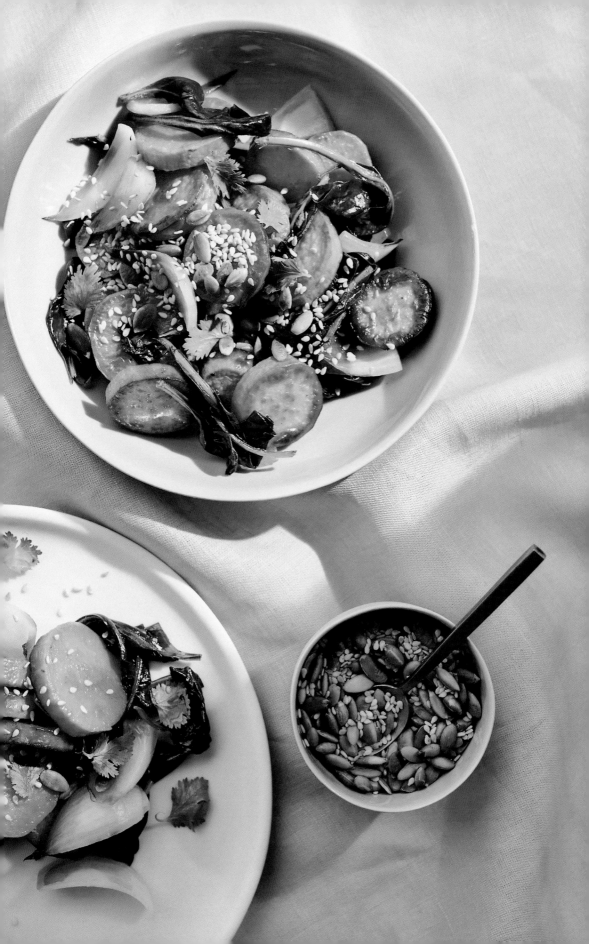

Roasted veggie stack

Serves: as many as you need · Prep: 10 minutes · Cook: 20 minutes

sweet potato

pumpkin

capsicum

zucchini

red onion

coconut oil spray

sea salt and freshly ground black pepper

balsamic glaze, to serve

hemp seeds, to serve

Preheat the oven to 180°C.

Slice all the veggies into long wide pieces.

Spray all the veggies with coconut oil and season with sea salt and freshly ground black pepper.

Line two baking trays with baking paper. Put the sweet potato and pumpkin on one tray and roast for 20 minutes.

Then lay the zucchini, onion and capsicum on a separate baking tray and roast for 15 minutes.

Once all the veggies are tender and cooked, layer them on a plate, starting with the sweet potato on the bottom.

Drizzle the balsamic glaze over the top, sprinkle with hemp seeds and enjoy!

Stuffed chicken

Serves: 1 · Prep: 5 minutes · Cook: 20 minutes

1 chicken breast

½ cup sun-dried tomatoes, sliced

1 handful of baby spinach leaves

15 g your choice of cheese, grated

3 tablespoons sauce of your choice (a good clean pasta sauce is good)

Preheat the oven to 180°C.

Using a very sharp knife, slice a deep pocket into the side of the chicken breast, without cutting all the way through.

Place the sun-dried tomato, spinach, cheese and sauce in the cavity.

Bake the chicken on a lined baking tray until cooked through; this should take about 20–30 minutes, so keep checking.

Serve warm. This is great with a side salad and some oven-baked sweet potato chips!

Raspberry cinnamon nice-cream

Serves: 1 · Prep: 10 minutes

1 cup frozen raspberries

5 tablespoons coconut yoghurt

1–2 teaspoons ground cinnamon

Put the raspberries in a bowl. Cover with the yoghurt, sprinkle with
the cinnamon and stir until the raspberries start to break down.

Put the bowl back in the freezer for 5 minutes before enjoying
as a quick, healthy dessert.

Blending the ingredients works well too;
if fully blended, you will need 15 minutes
in the freezer instead. You can also top with
cacao nibs for a crunchy texture.

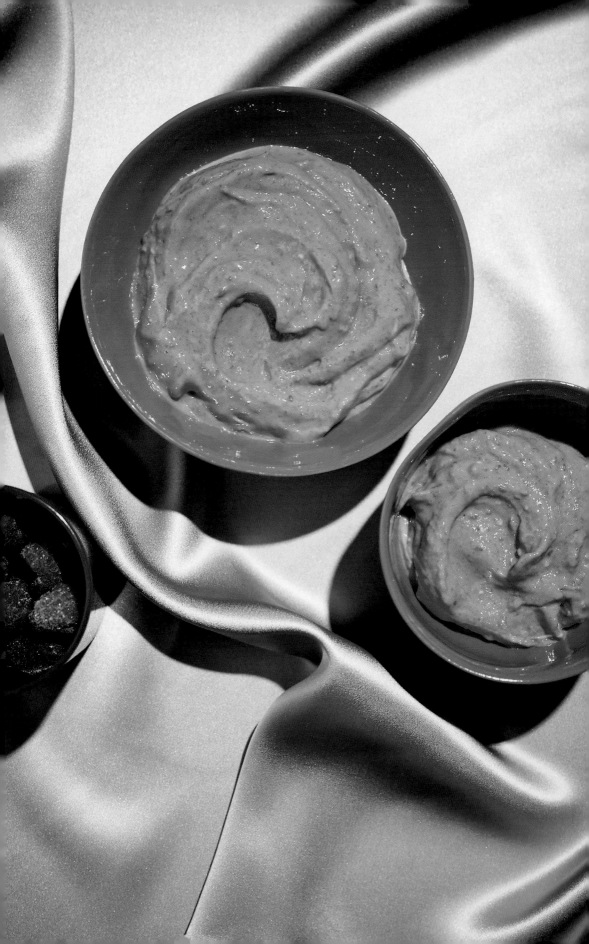

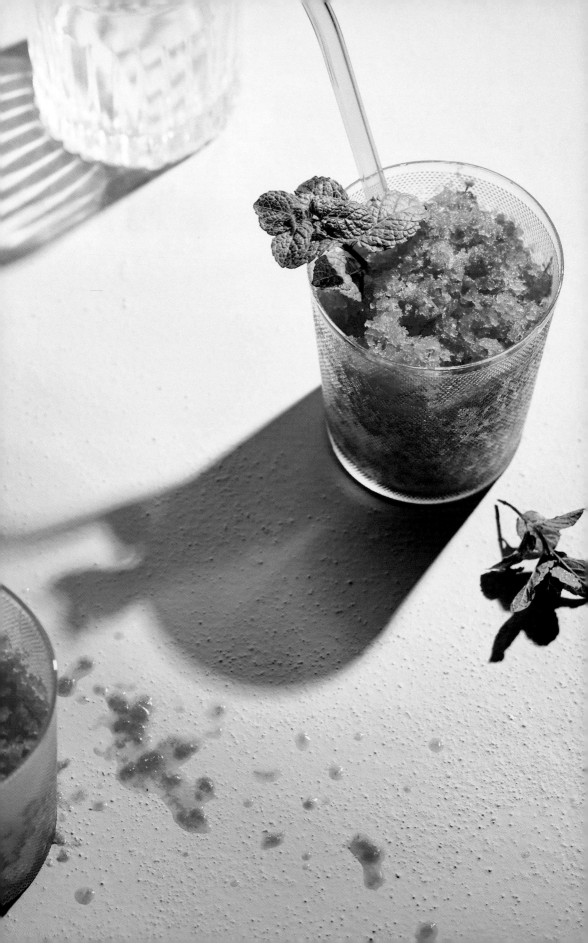

Mum's watermelon slushie

Serves: 4–6 · Prep: 10 minutes

1 large ripe watermelon

Lime juice

Mint leaves

Roughly chop the watermelon flesh and place it in a blender.

For every 3 cups of watermelon, add 2 tablespoons of lime juice, and 1–6 mint leaves, depending on your taste.

Blend for about 1 minute, until smooth. Pour into a shallow freezer dish and freeze for 1 hour.

Remove from the freezer and scrape the mixture with a fork, to start forming a slushie consistency.

Freeze for another 2 hours, then scrape the mixture again, to create a slushie or granita consistency. Once it is all icy goodness, you can serve!

If not eaten immediately, the mixture can be returned to the freezer, and scraped again before serving.

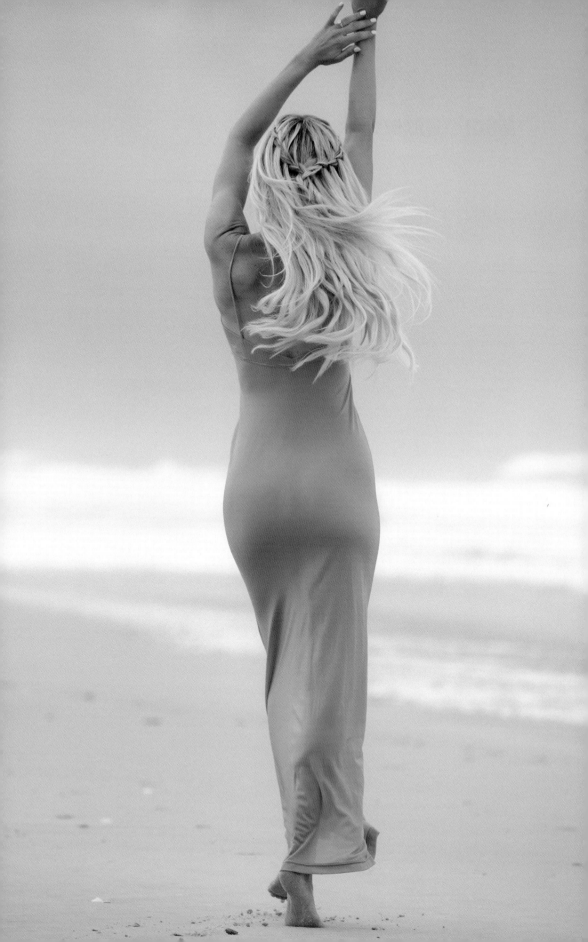

LESSON Fifteen

♥

It's ok to feel

WE *repeat* WHAT WE DON'T REPAIR

When I was growing up, my mum was really beautiful in letting me feel what I needed to feel. She never put pressure on me to be anything but myself and I'm so grateful to her.

However, there were people in my life whose voices stuck in my mind. I remember them saying things like…

Shhhhh!
Be quiet.
That's enough.
Stop crying.
That's not worth crying about.
That's silly.
You're being a sook.
No one wants to hear you blubbering.

I'm sure there may have been similar people in your life who responded to your emotions in a negative way and tried to shut them down.

If so, I'm SORRY that happened to you —
I know how that feels.

My real father actually didn't want to be a dad. From what I understand from my mum, he really wasn't ready for fatherhood, so when they mutually agreed the marriage wasn't working, he agreed to allow my mum full custody of us kids, and that was that.

On the very first date Mum had with my stepfather, he seemed like her dream man. At that stage, my mum was a very lonely, vulnerable, single mother of two young children. She certainly didn't have much support around her and was feeling very alone living out in the country.

I remember that first date, because my older brother and I went along too. He was extraordinary that day. He helped change a flat tyre for an elderly lady stuck on the side of the road. He actually saved my life at the beach that day when I fell into a massive deep hole in the ocean.

Understandably, he completely swept my mum off her feet. However, the honeymoon didn't last and the relationship deteriorated. It definitely wasn't the forever relationship mum had hoped to have.

In the end, Mum was so torn. She had zero self-worth. She so desperately didn't want another marriage to fall apart and she was determined that her family was going to stay together, no matter what. She so badly wanted to believe we could all somehow work this out.

Mum threw herself into work and put so much effort into being the best mum she could for us kids.

Eventually she was able to move on. We all needed to move on with our lives.

Ever since then, my mum, my brothers and I have been a strong family unit, and we are there for each other in every possible way.

Today, most of us are so very lucky to have the internet at our fingertips, giving us access to more knowledge, information and awareness about how we can do things better. Yes, the internet has its downsides, but the past decade has been amazing in creating a huge shift in the way people are feeling empowered to speak up more. They are finding their voices, and learning how to use them to express how they are feeling, they no longer feel ashamed if their marriage is falling apart.

Over time, I have come to see how family dynamics can have a big effect on our lives. I saw families go through really tough times when I was growing up. Often, marriages fail and the kids fall between the cracks. There can be physical abuse and emotional abuse – because the yelling and put downs can be just as bad. Often the adults were themselves abused as children, and pass it on without understanding the impact of their behaviour. I imagine that many parents believe that they are doing a good job with their children, but the children are in fact really suffering.

But boy oh boy, do I want to do the right thing with our little guy! Teaching Taj about all of his emotions and how to feel through them all is a priority for me as a mum. And as parents, Steve and I want to always provide a really safe space for Taj to express himself. Creating a family situation that is supportive and nourishing for everyone is a priority for Steve and me.

Although my husband recently turned 40, it's only in the past few years that I've really seen him open up and be honest when it comes to his feelings. It can be so hard for the men in our lives to express themselves and share their feelings, because of the ingrained macho, tough-guy stereotype, which hits back at them with comments like:

> *Don't cry, be a man! Don't be a pussy! Man up!*
> *Stop being a girl! Be a real man.*

Men can be very reluctant to talk about their feelings or show emotion, for fear of being seen as less masculine or of being accused of not being a 'real man'. This societal pressure encourages our men to remain quiet, to stay silent and to suppress their emotions, so that they end up dealing with them in unhealthy ways.

Suppressing and not expressing your feelings can lead you to turn to other things such as food, drugs, alcohol or even sex as a way to mask or numb your true feelings. Yes, it's true that it can be really painful to feel – but it's devastating that so many men have never learned a positive way to move through their emotions.

Drugs, alcohol and food can become a big distraction. I believe that if someone becomes addicted to these things, it's maybe because deep down there is a lot of hurt and deep wounds that have never healed. Feeling the full force and gamut of our own emotions can be so hard and uncomfortable that most of us want to just walk away from it, or metaphorically shove it under the rug, hoping it never resurfaces again!

A lot of the time, feelings hurt. They make us cry and make us feel uncomfortable.

But it is so important, necessary and better for us to feel through whatever comes up. While it's happening, it is critical for us to remember that thoughts are just thoughts – they will pass and won't last forever. By allowing our feelings to rise to the surface and finding the right tools to navigate through them, we will move through those feelings much faster – and in a much healthier way.

The sooner we really feel them, the sooner we can heal those wounds and truly be our true selves. It doesn't serve us to remain stuck in the past, surrounded by our traumas and triggers. That is in no way healthy.

It took me a very long time to acknowledge my feelings, without trying to outrun them or do my best to distract myself from thinking about them.

When I felt out of control with what was going on, it made me feel horrible and I would then aim to control other aspects of my life, such as food, training or people. But no matter how much I tried to distract myself and run from my feelings, I couldn't escape them – they would always, always resurface! In fact, the more I tried ignoring them, the harder it became to discuss them and start the healing process. Please don't do that to yourself – it just prolongs the pain.

FEELING THE FEELINGS

I want to share with you what I've learned to do – in the hope that it might help YOU, too.

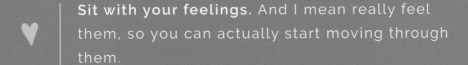

Sit with your feelings. And I mean really feel them, so you can actually start moving through them.

Cry! I do cry if I need to, or even scream into my pillow if it's all too much.

Sometimes I swim in the ocean. Do whatever is comfortable and healthy for you – remember you just need to do something to release all the feelings. Releasing feels good!

Speak to someone you trust. I love to reach out to my mentors, coaches, good friends, family and, of course, my husband. Staying silent and not getting support of some kind can really make me feel alone. None of us have to feel like that – there is always someone in our lives who will listen and care. For instance, Steve has a male coach who has such a great balance of masculine and feminine energy and has really helped Steve feel safe to be vulnerable and open to discussing so much.

Over the past decade, I've connected with so many incredible people who have helped me with so many different things I've struggled with, both mentally and emotionally. In this lesson, I'd like to acknowledge some of the people who have worked with me to make some big break-throughs and shifts in my life. Maybe, one day, if you're going through the same thing and are searching for help, they might be worth check-ing out. It may even be helpful for where you're at today – because, let's face it, we can never know enough! The more we know, the better we can do – and the better we become.

As I've mentioned previously, one of the massive influences in my life has been motivational coach Tony Robbins. He is responsi-ble for helping me to really understand myself, including my thought processes and my patterns of behaviour. His ability to break down human psychology to help us understand why we do the things we do is amazing. And I love that he also equips us with practical tools so that we can work our way through things. Tony Robbins has been life-changing for me.

Energy healer and counsellor Moira Williams is someone else who has helped me to work through a lot of my childhood wounds. Luckily for me, she is based on the Gold Coast in Queensland, where I live! Her focus is on dealing with unhealed childhood wounds and how they impact and affect us in our day-to-day lives, in our relationships and when we are faced with challenges. She was one of the key people who helped me get through a lot of wounds relating to my my biolog-ical father, my stepfather, and also the end of a friendship with one of my closest besties.

On my 'go to' list when I need 'No Bullshit' advice is Katie Dean. Not only is she a wellness coach and expert in managing and educat-ing people about anxiety, but she is also a good friend! This woman is fearless when it comes to truth-bombing absolutely anything – but it's always done with love. No matter what I reach out to talk about, there is zero judgement. I just love her!

The two coaches responsible for getting me through those six months of darkness when I was being viciously bullied online were Alexi Panos and Preston Smiles. Their guidance, support and coaching was invaluable. Together, they helped give me real insight, perspective and understanding about what was really going on. They helped me to heal old wounds and turned one of the biggest challenges of my life into an opportunity for growth.

Okay, just one more … relationship coach Bryan Reeves. This man has really helped change and shape my relationship with my husband Steve SO much over the past few years. One of the greatest things has been to make Steve feel safe to be vulnerable and not just talk about things but to be able to cry. This makes sense when you know Steve's dad passed away when Steve was just 12 years old. From that moment on, Steve had to step up and be 'the man' of the family, taking on the responsibility of looking after everyone around him. This has been the first time Steve has had that backup, support and deep level of understanding from another male since he lost his father. Our relationship together has also grown so much stronger as a result of the work Steve has been doing with Bryan. We are way more connected and have a deeper sense of compassion and understanding of each other's struggles, needs and wants. The vision of what our ultimate relationship and life together could look like is much clearer. We have a lot of coaching sessions together as a couple, but also each of us has one-on-one sessions with Bryan as well. We've learned to not wait until we feel we need a session, but schedule them in regularly so that we always have an outlet to discuss anything that might be showing up for us or that we might be struggling to work through alone.

Even as adults, so many of us carry childhood wounds that show up in our daily lives. We can't ignore them. As hard as it is, we have to talk about them and move through them. Addressing old wounds opens up the possibility for us to not just heal – but to GROW! The added benefit is how much lighter you will feel, because it literally feels like a weight has been lifted off your shoulders. It allows us to stop spending valuable energy and time on those old wounds and instead refocus on things that make us feel great!

Why would you let the past hold you back from being the greatest version of yourself that you can possibly BE?

MY TOP 10 LIFE LESSONS

Now that you've finished reading about the 15 Life Lessons that have really helped me, I'd love it if you could please take some time to write down the 10 lessons that have really vibed with you!

10 THINGS I WANT TO CHANGE OR DO DIFFERENTLY IN MY LIFE

1 |

2 |

3 |

4 |

5 |

6 |

7 |

8 |

9 |

10 |

CONVERSION CHART

Measuring cups and spoons may vary slightly from one country to another, but the difference is generally not enough to affect a recipe. All cup and spoon measures are level.

One Australian metric measuring cup holds 250 ml (8 fl oz), one Australian tablespoon holds 20 ml (4 teaspoons) and one Australian metric teaspoon holds 5 ml. North America, New Zealand and the UK use a 15 ml (3-teaspoon) tablespoon.

LENGTH

METRIC	IMPERIAL
3 mm	⅛ inch
6 mm	¼ inch
1 cm	½ inch
2.5 cm	1 inch
5 cm	2 inches
18 cm	7 inches
20 cm	8 inches
23 cm	9 inches
25 cm	10 inches
30 cm	12 inches

LIQUID MEASURES

ONE AMERICAN PINT	ONE IMPERIAL PINT
500 ml (16 fl oz)	600 ml (20 fl oz)

CUP	METRIC	IMPERIAL
⅛ cup	30 ml	1 fl oz
¼ cup	60 ml	2 fl oz
⅓ cup	80 ml	2½ fl oz
½ cup	125 ml	4 fl oz
⅔ cup	160 ml	5 fl oz
¾ cup	180 ml	6 fl oz
1 cup	250 ml	8 fl oz
2 cups	500 ml	16 fl oz
2¼ cups	560 ml	20 fl oz
4 cups	1 litre	32 fl oz

DRY MEASURES

METRIC	IMPERIAL
15 g	½ oz
30 g	1 oz
60 g	2 oz
125 g	4 oz (¼ lb)
185 g	6 oz
250 g	8 oz (½ lb)
375 g	12 oz (¾ lb)
500 g	16 oz (1 lb)
1 kg	32 oz (2 lb)

OVEN TEMPERATURES

CELSIUS	FAHRENHEIT
100°C	200°F
120°C	250°F
150°C	300°F
160°C	325°F
180°C	350°F
200°C	400°F
220°C	425°F

CELSIUS	GAS MARK
110°C	¼
130°C	½
140°C	1
150°C	2
170°C	3
180°C	4
190°C	5
200°C	6
220°C	7
230°C	8
240°C	9
250°C	10

ACKNOWLEDGEMENTS

Thank you just doesn't feel like a strong enough word to express my deep gratitude to you ALL for supporting my journey. You've read every post, watched each Snapchat or YouTube video and now you're reading this book. Along the way you've let me help you raise your own baseline to live a happier, healthier life so you too can achieve your dreams. Being brave enough to dive into this book to reflect on life and on yourself shows your commitment to being the best possible version of you.

To my whole team for backing me every step of the way, believing in me and reminding me that what I have to say matters. Our combined goals and vision in wanting to make a difference in the world, especially for women, is so aligned.

To Levi, I've admired you for years. You've always believed in me and my mission to stand tall and to be proud of who I am. You're also the one responsible for helping me to understand more about myself and my health, which has allowed me to share this knowledge with so many other women.

To Renata, for pushing me and believing in me when I kept saying 'No, I can't write a book.' For your commitment to the work, LONG hours and days, your invaluable experience and eye for detail, your creativity and wanting everything to be nothing short of amazing. Your dedication to your work and passion for bringing this to life is something I'm so grateful for.

To Taylor, the way you throw yourself in the deep end and just go for it is so inspiring. Together we create magic and always have the same vision when it comes to anything creative. I love all of your input, images, ideas and commitment to me as a person and my whole brand. We're so aligned with what we want for each project and this book is something you too should be proud of.

To Kelsea, thanks for being my right hand through everything and anything these past few years. No matter what the task, you show up and do it with such grace and professionalism. You're there for me through all my good and bad days. I appreciate so much the final touches and effort you put into making sure everything runs smoothly.

To Carlotta, you have a way to make me feel so comfortable in front of the camera and from the very first shot you allowed me to just be me. The images are everything I wanted and more.

To Jasmine and Kristy, my glam team and the BEST hair and make-up artists in the business. It's incredible how fast you work but your hair and make-up talent is something else! Thank you for coming on this ride with me and bringing out the best in my looks for the book. Love you both!

To my beautiful mum for loving me endlessly and unconditionally. Although we were thrown some challenges I always knew how much you loved me and you've always shown up for me no matter what. There's nothing I'd change about you and I cannot thank you enough for being my rock, my best friend and the best mum in the world. You are everything.

My darling little man Taj, you have been one of my biggest teachers and you give me a whole new purpose in life. Every single day you make me want to be better than I was yesterday. I want to be your inspiration and biggest rock so you know I'll have your back no matter what. Thank you for being an all-round bloody legend of a human and the sweetest boy I've ever known, with the biggest heart. You don't realise it now – but you are one of the biggest drivers for everything that I do. I want this world to be a better place for you and I won't ever stop being there for you and everyone who needs me.

Last but DEF not least – to my loving, supportive and incredibly encouraging husband, Steve. When we first met I didn't believe in myself at all – not one bit. But you always saw something in me and pushed me, encouraged me and pushed me some more to chase my dreams of helping women find happiness, health and confidence in every area of their life. I owe it ALL to you for believing in me. I don't think I ever would ever have tried making something of myself without you by my side.

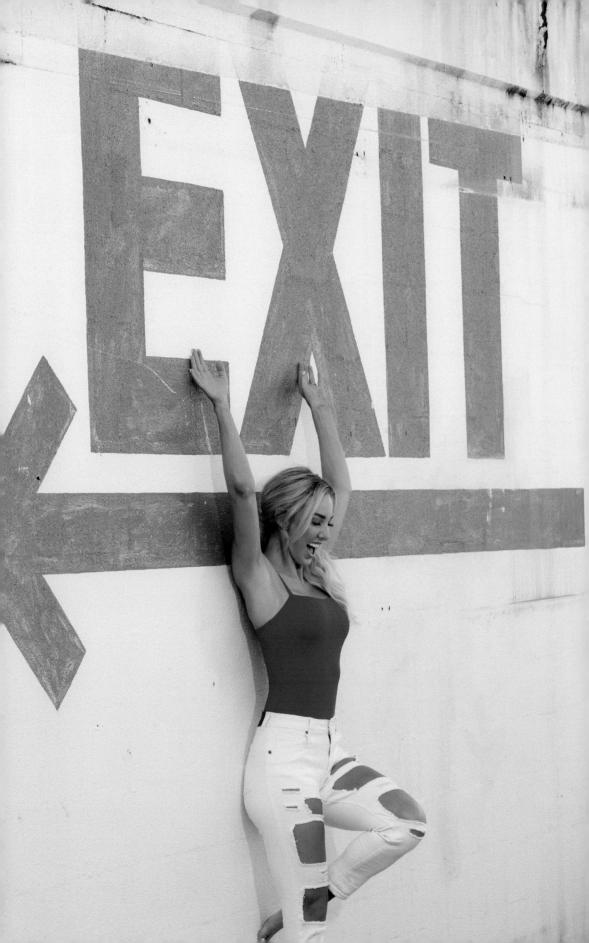

First published 2020 in Macmillan
by Pan Macmillan Australia Pty Limited
Level 25, 1 Market Street, Sydney, New South Wales
Australia 2000

A CIP catalogue record for this book is available from the National Library of Australia:
http://catalogue.nla.gov.au

Design by Taylor Peet with Alissa Dinallo
Edited by Katri Hilden
Editorial & Creative Director, Ashy Bines Group, Renata Gombac
Prop and food styling by Lynsey Fryers
Food preparation by Tamika O'Neill
Hair by Kristy Gibson
Makeup by Jasmine Lei Creations

Many thanks to Light Years Diner in Burleigh Heads and The Dusty Road for their furniture upholstery.

Colour + reproduction by Splitting Image Colour Studio
Printed in China by Imago Printing International Limited

10 9 8 7 6 5 4 3 2 1